Case Studies of Near Misses in Clinical Anesthesia

John G. Brock-Utne

Case Studies of Near Misses in Clinical Anesthesia

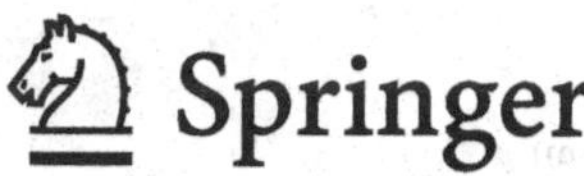

John G. Brock-Utne, MD, PhD, FFA(SA)
Professor of Anesthesia
Stanford University Medical Center
Stanford, CA 94305-5640, USA
brockutn@stanford.edu

ISBN 978-1-4419-1178-0 e-ISBN 978-1-4419-1179-7
DOI 10.1007/978-1-4419-1179-7
Springer New York Dordrecht Heidelberg London

Library of Congress Control Number: 2011931890

Printed on acid-free paper

Springer is part of Springer Science+Business Media (www.springer.com)

For the next generation:

Matthew B. Brock-Utne
Tobias J. Brock-Utne
Anders C. Brock-Utne
Jasper L. Brock-Utne
Stefan S. Brock-Utne

Foreword

The anesthetic care of most of our patients often seems routine. For the majority, a preoperative evaluation management plan is made and followed, and the anesthesia and surgery proceeds as planned. Anesthesiologists do not like surprises! But, sometimes (and thankfully not often) the case does not follow the script, and unanticipated events occur. Patients have idiosyncratic responses to medications, or experience surgical or anesthetic misadventures that lead to changes in vital signs or worse. These events are few and far between, and if you have not witnessed them previously, you might not consider some of the more unusual causes for these presentations. John Brock-Utne has once again collected a series of such "rare" events. Each case discussion considers the presentation, his diagnosis, and then his approach to management. In each instance, catastrophe was avoided. Every case in this book is real, and similar events could occur tomorrow to patients under the care of the reader. It is the early recognition of these "near miss" episodes and the "lessons learned" in managing them that make this book so important. Dr. Brock-Utne's many years of experience, his interesting way of presenting the case scenarios, and his practical no-frills approach to management make this book a must-read. My own anesthetic practice, that of my colleagues at Stanford University, and the hundreds of anesthesia residents who have come through our program over the past three decades have all benefitted from knowing and working with Dr. Brock-Utne. This book allows others to learn from his experiences.

Stanford, CA

Jay B. Brodsky, MD

Preface

As anesthesiologists we are confronted, from time to time, with difficult decisions in "near miss" situations. Fortunately, "near misses" occur rarely, but it is important to be aware that they can occur. This book is a companion to my previous book *Clinical Anesthesia: Near Misses and Lessons Learned*, published by Springer in 2008. That book also described "near misses." The cases in this book are all new. Together these books relate to my 41 years of clinical anesthesia experience in Scandinavia, South Africa, and the United States.

Each of the 80 cases gives the reader, on the first page, all the information necessary to diagnose/treat a potential disaster. The next page provides solution(s) and a discussion of the problem(s), makes recommendations, and provides references, where appropriate, for further reading.

The suggested management of these cases may be controversial. If so, they may form the basis for a teaching discussion between faculty members and residents/fellows-in-training in anesthesiology. But most of all, this book is designed to alert the reader to various precarious situations that can arise in anesthesia practice in both sophisticated and rural anesthetic environments and how to best prevent or deal with them. To paraphrase Goethe:

> The art is long,
> Life is short;
> Experiment perilous,
> Decisions difficult.

After all these years in anesthesia, I can honestly say Goethe was right.

Stanford, CA, USA　　　John G. Brock-Utne, MD, PhD, FFA(SA)

Acknowledgments

I would like to acknowledge my many colleagues around the world who have contributed to this book through case discussions and/or case reports:

Aileen Adriano, Scott Ahlbrand, Dondee Almazan, Sid J. Aidines, John Aitchison, Tim Angelotti, Martin Angst, Dave Armstrong, Dan Azar, Rob Becker, Jonathan Bradley, Marisa Brandt, Pat Bolton, Greg Botz, Ioana Brisc, Arne J. Brock-Utne, Jay B. Brodsky, Michael Brook, Carlos Brun, Alex Butwick, Brendan Carvalho, Jorge A. Caballero, Michael Charles, Michael Chen, Sheila Cohen, Lawrence Chu, Peter S. Chard, Michael Charles, John L. Chow, Rebecca Claure, Jeremy Collins, Tara Cornaby, John Cummings, Matt R. Eng, Jay Jay Desai, Alimorad Djalali, Anthony Doufas, Laura Downey, David Drover, Joshua Edwards, Terje Eide, Roy Esaki, William Feaster, Steve Fisher, Maika Fujiki, Mark Gjolai, Eric Gross, Cosmin Guta, Ali Habibi, Gordon Haddow, Jennifer Hah, T. Kyle Harrison, Erin Hennessy, J. Hester, Gill Hilton, Alan Hold, John S. Ikonomidis, Jerry Ingrande, Richard A. Jaffe, Matthew Jolley, Jack Kan, Andrew Kim, Matthew Kolz, Elliot Krane, Vivek Kulkarni, Shaun Kunnavatana, Merlin Larsson, Gary Lau, Jennifer Lee, David Levi, Richard M. Levitan, Harry J.M. Lemmens, Geoff Lighthall, Steve Lipman, Paul Lukin, Alex Macario, Sean Mackey, Rajend Maharaj, Kevin Malott, Jim B.D. Mark, Richard Mazze, Diana McGregor, Fred Mihm, Brett Miller, Samuel Mireles, Vanessa Moll, John Morton, Rai Naidu, Sim Naiker, Andrew Neice, John Nguyen, Mohammed Omar, Einar Ottestad, David Parris, Ron Pearl, Catherine Reid, Periklis Panousis, Fred J. Pinto, Frain Rivera, Beemeth Robles, Myer Rosenthal, Edward Riley, George K. Roberts, John Probst, Lawrence Saidman, Carolyn Schifftner, Cliff Schmiesing, Ingela Schnittger, Vikas Shah, Larry C. Siegel, Vanilla Sing, Øyvind Skraastad, David Soran, Kjell Erik Stroemskag, Naiyi Sun, John Talvera, Pedro Tanaka, Gordon Taylor, Ying Tian, Ankeet Udani, Pieter van der Starre, Lindsey Vokach-Brodsky, Kimberly Valenta, Mark Vierra, Tracy Vogel, Richard Whyte, Becky Wong, Jimmy Wong, Bernhard Wranne, Troy T. Wu, Karl Zheng, Andy A. Zumaran, and Imad M. Yamout.

I am also greatly indebted to the following people:

Dr. Jay B. Brodsky, who kindly agreed to write a foreword for this book. Besides being a wonderful friend, he is also a superb clinical anesthesiologist, clinical researcher, and organizer of the operating room at Stanford. The Stanford University Department of Anesthesia is indeed fortunate to have such an outstanding physician.

Bernadett Mahanay, my secretary in the Department of Anesthesia Stanford University School of Medicine, for her unfailing good humor and tremendous dedication to her job. Without her willingness to help, I doubt there would have been a sequel.

To the many, many residents, with whom I have had the pleasure to be involved in their anesthesia training. I am extremely grateful for all their challenging and stimulating questions, their enthusiasm for anesthesia, and for many hours of thoughtful discussion.

Joanna Perey and Shelley Reinhardt, both of Springer, for all their hard work, support, and encouragement.

Last but not least, my wife Sue, our boys, Jens, Arne, and Ivar, their wives Alice and Jennifer, and our five grandsons: Matthew, Tobias, Anders, Jasper, and Stefan.

Stanford, CA, USA John G. Brock-Utne, MD, PhD, FFA(SA)

Contents

Chapter 1
Case 1: A Patient with a Mediastinal Mass

Today you are an attending anesthesiologist in a large university medical center. The first case is a 55-year-old gentleman (60 kg, 5 ft 11 in.) with multiple metastatic melanomas. He has had one metastasis removed from his brain in the past. He now presents with some speech impairment and is scheduled for a tumor resection close to his speech center. His past history is significant for a difficult airway, hypertension, and coronary artery disease. A previous anesthesia record from another hospital informs you that the patient had a grade 4 view. The airway was, at that time, secured by using a bougie. His coronary artery disease is stated to be stable. He is 90 kg and is 6 ft 1 in. tall. You arrange for an awake fiberoptic cart to be available in the morning.

On the day of surgery, you review the chart and find to your dismay that he also has a mediastinal mass at the level of the carina. Four months ago the mass was approximately 4 cm in diameter. The mass was 3 cm on a previous investigation. The date of the earlier investigation is not stated. The tumor is situated behind the carina. A bronchoscopy, performed 4 months ago, shows a constriction at the origin of the right main bronchus. The lumen being 80% obstructed for 1–2 cm. No investigation has been done since then. He has no breathing problem, no shortness of breath, orthopnea, coughing, wheezing, stridor, and hematopoiesis. On examination he is a lying with two pillows under his head on the gurney in the preoperative area. His vital signs are stable and his oxygen saturation is 98% on room air. He has no problem lying flat or sitting up. Since he is unsteady on his feet, he does not exercise. His laboratory values are within normal limits. No arterial blood gas has been done.

You consider canceling the case and get a new scan and a new bronchoscopy. However, the surgeon is concerned that if we delay, the tumor's involvement of the speech center may progress to such an extent that it may not be possible to remove the tumor without damaging the speech center. In view of that you call in a pulmonologist and take the patient to the OR. Under sedation with midazolam and

J.G. Brock-Utne, *Case Studies of Near Misses in Clinical Anesthesia*,
DOI 10.1007/978-1-4419-1179-7_1,

topical lidocaine 4%, the pulmonologist performs a fiberoptic bronchoscopy. The findings are now much worse than before. The lower trachea from the carina is obstructed by about 80%. The length of the obstruction is 5 cm. The finding in the right main bronchus remains unchanged, while the left bronchus was found to be normal. The tissue in the trachea is normal with no bleeding or erosions.

Questions

What would you do now? Cancel the case? Would you proceed and if so how?

Solution

This case happened to me. I felt that since the patient was asymptomatic, from his respiratory point of view and by hopefully saving his speech center from tumor involvement, we went ahead. The pulmonologist, at my suggestion, had already got a #8 endotracheal tube (ETT) "loaded" on the scope. When the decision was made to proceed, the ETT was placed in the trachea without any problem. The cuff was inflated in the upper trachea without involving the tumor that was bulging into the posterior aspect of the trachea. This was verified by the fiberoptic scope. The airway pressures were never more than 19 cm H_2O, and the airway loop was normal. At the end of the surgery, with the patient breathing spontaneously, a tube changer was placed into the patient's ETT and the ETT removed. The tube changer was placed in the airway, in this difficult airway patient, so that you can easily secure the airway should trachea collapse after the ETT was removed. After the ETT was removed, the patient was seen to breathe without any problem and the tube changer was removed. In the OR, he was able to move all limbs and his vital signs were normal. The patient was taken to the ICU for postoperative care. He was discharged home 3 days later with an appointment to see his oncologist for further evaluations.

Recommendation

At times you must weigh all the pros and cons. In this case I would say we were lucky.

References

1. Berth U, Lichtor JL. Anterior mediastinal mass. Anesthesiology. 2010;112:447.
2. Prackash UB, Abel MD, Hubmayr RD. Mediastinal mass and tracheal obstruction during general anesthesia. Mayo Clin Proc. 1998;63:1004–11.
3. Erdos G, Tzanova I. Perioperative anesthesia management of mediastinal masses in adults. Eur J Anaesthesiol. 2009;26:627–32.
4. Bechard P, Letourneau L, Lacasse Y, Cote D, Bussieres JS. Perioperative cardiorespiratory complications in adults with medistinal mass: incidence and risk factors. Anesthesiology. 2004;100:826–34.

Solution

References

Chapter 2
Case 2: Stick Out Your Tongue

As an "el toro" anesthesiologist in Oslo, Norway in 1970, I watched with interest a visiting Australian anesthesiologist (Dr. Sid J. Aidinis) waking up patients. At the end of every anesthetic, after the endotracheal tube was removed, he would say in Norwegian: "Stikk ut tongen din" (Stick out your tongue). The patient if awake enough would always oblige. I asked him: "Why don't you just ask him to squeeze your hand?" He looked at me and said:

There are several reasons for why you want the patient to stick out their tongue at the end of a general anesthetic:

1. The patient shows that he/she can follow a command. Of course you could get the same answer with squeezing your hand, but there are more reasons.
2. The patient indicates that he/she can protect their airway. This is something hand squeezing can't do.
3. Early studies on clinical monitoring of the neuromuscular function have suggested that protruding the tongue is a good assessment of return of neuromuscular function [1].
4. Sticking out your tongue is a very unusual request. It would be highly unlikely for someone to stick out their tongue unless asked to do so. Furthermore, squeezing your hand has a higher chance of happening by chance than protruding the tongue would.
5. The 12 cranial nerve is intact (a minor point) but there is another reason which is probably the most important one of all. Can you, John, tell me what that is?

Question

I could not and now I ask you, the reader, to come up with the answer. What do you think the other reason is?

J.G. Brock-Utne, *Case Studies of Near Misses in Clinical Anesthesia*,
DOI 10.1007/978-1-4419-1179-7_2, © Springer Science+Business Media, LLC 2011

Solution

Sid said:

> When the patient sticks his/her tongue, at your request, at the end of an anesthetic this is something you and everyone in the room can see. Hence, in a court of law, everyone in the operating room saw that the patient was awake and was following command at the end of the surgery. Remember that the patient squeezing your hand is something ONLY you can feel.

Recommendation

Asking your patient to stick the tongue out is a quick way to establish if the patient is awake and is following commands. It may also be a good measure of return of adequate muscle strength [2, 3]. But the most important reason is related to the fact that everyone can concur that this patient was awake at the end of the anesthetic.

In my anesthetic practice, I always ask my patients to stick their tongue out. When they do, it gives me great comfort.

References

1. Ali HH, Savarese JJ. Monitoring of neuormuscular function. Anesthesiology. 1976;45: 216–49.
2. Kopman AF. Neuromuscular monitoring: old issues, new controversies. J Clin Care. 2009;24: 11–20.
3. Murphy GS, Szokol JW, Marymont JH, Franklin M, Avram MJ, Vender JS. Resiudal paralysis at the time of tracheal extubation. Anesth Analg. 2005;100:1840–5.

Chapter 3
Case 3: An Epidural Blood Patch – What Went Wrong?

A 27-year-old woman para 2 (86 kg and 161 cm) had an accidental dural puncture at L3–4 spinal interspace during placement of an epidural for labor pain. The next attempt at L2–3 interspace was successful and the epidural analgesia for labor and delivery worked very well. She was discharged home with her baby 2 days later.

Three days later, she is back in the emergency room complaining of severe postdural-puncture headache. She agrees to a blood patch. The patient is placed in the lateral decubitus position and the epidural space located at L3–4 interspace using a loss of resistance to air technique. This is followed by 3 mL of 3% 2-chloroprocaine test dose. A bilateral sensor loss at T10–12 with no motor deficit is seen within 6 min. Thereafter, 20 mL of autologous blood is withdrawn in a sterile manner from the patient. The blood is injected through the epidural needlc and the needle removed. The patient is turned to the supine position. However within 2 min, she complains of shortness of breath. She is made to sit up. Sitting, you see she is using her accessory upper respiratory muscles. Her vital signs are the following: heart rate 68 bpm, BP is 88/50 mmHg, Oxygen saturation 96%, and respiratory rate 30. She has a sensory loss from C5 to S5 bilaterally. Her hand grip is weak. She is transferred to the postanesthesia care unit for observation. An hour later, she has recovered completely and much to her relief the headache has gone too. She is discharged home after having been in the hospital for 4 h.

Question

Why did she suddenly have difficulty in breathing?

J.G. Brock-Utne, *Case Studies of Near Misses in Clinical Anesthesia*,
DOI 10.1007/978-1-4419-1179-7_3, © Springer Science+Business Media, LLC 2011

Solution

This complication has been reported [1]. It is hypothesized that some of the local anesthetic entered the subarachnoid space via the previous dural puncture during the injection of the blood patch [2, 3]. It is also possible that the test dose was forced into the subarachnoid space by the blood patch without going through the dural puncture hole but just through the subarachnoid lining. This latter is a strong possibility. When you inject air into the epidural space during the loss of resistance technique, it has been shown that drugs and air can have unexpected easy access to the venous circulation and potentially also the subarachnoid space, producing potentially unwanted systemic effects [4].

Cohen and Amar [5] suggest that verifying the correct position of the epidural needle, prior to a blood patch, should be done with the gravity technique. This consists of an IV extension tubing filled with saline being attached to the epidural needle. The needle is in the correct position if the fluid level fluctuates with each heart beat. Cohen and Negron [1] further suggest that blood patching should be delayed until the patient is completely recovered from the neuraxial test dose block.

Total spinal anesthesia has also been reported following early prophylactic epidural blood patch done before the effects of the epidural lidocaine have worn off [2]. Furthermore the injection of saline into the epidural space, to hasten the speed of return of motor function [6, 7], has also been reported as causing a total spinal anesthesia [8].

Recommendation

It seems reasonable to recommend that no blood patch or fluid should be administered into the epidural space before the effects of any local anesthetic have worn off.

References

1. Cohen S, Negron M. A near total spinal anesthetic following a test dose prior to an epidural blood patch. Anesth Analg. 2008;107:727–8.
2. Leivers D. Total spinal anesthesia following early prophylactic epidural blood patch. Anesthesiology. 1990;73:1287.
3. Park PC, Berry PD, Larson MD. Total spinal anesthesia following epidural saline injection after prolonged epidural anesthesia. Anesthesiology. 1988;89:1267–70.
4. Jaffe RA, Siegel LC, Schnittger I, Propst JW, Brock Utne JG. Epidural air injection assessed by tranesophageal echocardiography. Reg Anesth. 1995;20:152–5.
5. Cohen S, Amar D. Epidural block for obstetrics: compression of bolus injection of local anesthestic with gravity flow technique. J Clin Anesth. 1997;9:623–8.

6. Johnson MD, Burger GA, Mushlin PS, Arthur GR, Datta S. Reversal of bupivacaine epidural anesthesia by intermittent epidural injections of crystalloid solutions. Anesth Analg. 1990; 70:393–9.
7. Brock-Utne JG, Macario A, Dillingham MF, Fanton GS. Postoperative epidural injection of saline can shorten postanesthesia care unit time for knee arthroscopy. Reg Anesth Pain Med. 1998;23:247–51.
8. Park PC, Berry P, Larson M. Total spinal anesthesia following epidural saline injection after prolonged epidural anesthesia. Anesthesiology. 1998;89:1267–70.

Chapter 4
Case 4: A Lack of Communication Leads to a Bad Outcome

You have just started your new job as an anesthesiologist. It is Saturday morning, and a 76-year-old man is scheduled for pinning of his fractured left hip. He is an inpatient having been admitted the evening before. You meet the patient (5 ft 11 in. and 75 kg) in the preoperative area. He fell down some stairs the previous afternoon, was taken to the hospital and admitted for surgery this morning. The patient is accompanied by his daughter-in-law and his son. His past medical history tells you that he is being treated for high blood pressure and hyperlipidemia. He has occasional heartburn for which he takes Mylanta. His vital signs are stable. You exam him and find no other injuries and his chest is clear. He has not eaten since lunchtime the previous day. You review the hospitalist note who informs you that he has been vomiting in the night but this was thought to be due to meperidine that had been given to him in the ER. He had been prescribed an antiemetic with good result. The patient says that he does not feel nauseous now and that he has not vomited for hours. His Hct is 36% and the basic metabolic panel is normal. You give him an ASA 2 rating.

You suggest a spinal anesthetic with the possibility of a general anesthetic if the spinal does not work. He and the family agree and the consent is signed. You sedate him with 1 mg of midazolam and perform a "one-shot femoral" nerve block on the left side [1]. He is brought to the operating room and you give him Bicitra 30 mL per os. With the patient sitting up on the gurney, you attempt a spinal block. Unfortunately after 10–15 min, you give up as you can't get into the intrathecal space. The patient is gently positioned supine and you perform a rapid sequence induction with cricoids pressure. As you open his mouth, a large amount of "coffee ground" emesis come up into the oropharynx. While the assistant continues to hold cricoids pressure, you put the patient in Trendelenburg and suck the oropharynx clean. Thereafter, you place an endotracheal tube (ETT) in his trachea and suction the ETT prior to commencing ventilation. To your dismay you obtain a lot of "coffee ground" fluid from suctioning down the ETT. You reevaluate the patient's vital signs

J.G. Brock-Utne, *Case Studies of Near Misses in Clinical Anesthesia*,
DOI 10.1007/978-1-4419-1179-7_4, © Springer Science+Business Media, LLC 2011

and find that his peek pressures are 25 cm H_2O, his oxygen saturation is 99%, and his heart rate and blood pressure are within normal limits.

Questions

What will you do now? Cancel the case? Proceed? What is this brownish fluid anyway? The surgeon mentions that we better proceed with the surgery otherwise the patient will get a compartment syndrome of his thigh. Is this a concern?

Solution

This happened to a friend of mine. He decides to carry on with the operation. The "coffee ground" fluid was sent to the laboratory. Forty minutes later it was confirmed as heme. You now suspect a stress ulcer and you order an ICU bed for the patient. The operation is concluded after 2 h and the patient is taken to the ICU. Unfortunately, he develops adult respiratory distress syndrome and after 6 weeks in the ICU, the patient dies.

My friend later establishes that the patient had hemoptysis several times during the night prior to surgery. In fact the total amount was over 1,000 mL from midnight to 6 a.m. This was faithfully recorded by the nursing staff. The nurses had told the surgeon about the "coffee ground" emesis, on the morning of the day of surgery. Hearing this, the surgeon rang the hospitalist who had just come on duty. The hospitalist, without seeing the patient and just read the notes, said: "Yes, he is cleared for surgery." No one told the anesthesiologist, not even the son who had been in the room all night with the patient, that coffee ground emesis had been observed. It is of interest to note that there was no evidence of emesis on the patient's bed sheets or his pajamas when he came down for surgery accompanied by a ward nurse. That was because the patient and sheets were all cleaned up after every emesis.

This case is an example of a total breakdown of communication between nurses, hospitalist, surgeon, and the anesthesiologist. After the death of the patient, his son took the surgeon, hospitalist, the hospital, and the anesthesiologist to court. My friend was found innocent, but the hospital was found guilty.

Recommendations

Recommendations in this case are several:

1. Should one ask the color of the vomit every time a patient tells you that he or she has vomited? No, one would hope that most people would tell you the color of the vomit. Had my friend been informed, he would have canceled the case and asked a gastroenterologist to see the patient urgently.
2. Compartment syndrome. Although serious, in the thigh region it is very unlikely as the thigh is not like the lower leg which is defined by muscle and fascial compartments. I don't think there has been a case reported of compartment syndrome in the thigh following hip fracture.
3. I always make a point of asking the surgeon when they book an emergency case: "Is there anything you think that I may want to know about this patient?" You be surprised how often they remember things that may not be in the notes, but are of great importance to the welfare of the patient.

Reference

1. Brock-Utne JG. Clinical anesthesia. Near misses and lessons learnt page. New York: Springer; 2008. p. 10–1.

Chapter 5
Case 5: Hyperkalemia During Coronary Artery Bypass Graft

A 76-year-old male (5 ft 8 in. and 82 kg) is scheduled for a three vessel CABG and Aortic valve replacement. His past history is significant for three vessel CAD (70% LAD, 70 Circ, and 70% RCA). The aortic stenostic valve area is 0.69 cm^2 and the gradient is 36 mmHg. The patient also has chronic renal insufficiency with a (Cr) of 1.4–1.9 in the past year. He also is a non-insulin diabetic and has obstructive sleep apnea. Surgery is now indicated because of increased shortness of breath on minimal exercise. His medication was gemfibrozil, amitriptyline, aspirin, HCTZ, and atenolol. On physical exam, you find a cardiac murmur at right upper sternal border radiating to the carotids. The lungs are clear and EKG shows NSR with no ischemic changes. The ECHO shows an ejection fraction of 55–60%. The laboratory values are within normal levels with a K of 4.4 mmol/L, but the Cr is 1.4.

Rapid sequence induction is performed in a routine manner using fentanyl 500 mcg, etomidate 12 mg, and rocuronium 100 mg. An endotracheal tube, PA catheter, and a TEE are all placed successfully. As per surgeon's request, Epsilon-Aminocaproic Acid (Amicar) 5 g is started IV in a dose of 1 g/h at 8:20 a.m. The patient's vital sign remains stable. Fifty-five minutes into the case, a routine arterial blood gas (ABG) reveals a K of 5.5 mmol/L. Fifteen minutes later, a repeat ABG shows the K to have increased to 6.4 mmol/L. You note that the urine output has been 200 mL since the start of surgery. The amount of IV NaCl is 1,200 mL. No potassium or blood products have been given. The blood sugar is normal.

Question

What will you do and what can be the problem?

J.G. Brock-Utne, *Case Studies of Near Misses in Clinical Anesthesia*,
DOI 10.1007/978-1-4419-1179-7_5,

Solution

Slowly administer calcium chloride 500 mg and frusemide 5 mg, 10 units of IV insulin, and one ampoule of 50% dextrose solution. One hour later the K is 4.6 mmol/L.

There are at least two cases reporting an increase in serum K after the infusion of Amicar [1, 2]. One case [2] was so refractory to the above treatment, including 30 mg of polystyrene sulphonate (kayexalate) as a retention enema that the patient had to be treated with hemodialysis.

The acute increase in serum potassium most likely resulted from a shift of potassium from the intracellular space to the extracellular space. The acute increase in serum potassium could not be explained by either an excessive input of potassium or a primary failure of renal potassium excretions. There was no clinical or laboratory evidence for hemolysis or rhabdomyolysis. Furthermore, severe thrombocytosis or leukocytoses were not present making pseudohyperkalemia an unlikely cause of the increased potassium. Insulinopenia with impaired cellular uptake of potassium was unlikely since the plasma glucose was normal. Since succinylcholine was not used, this could not be the cause of the increase in potassium.

Recommendation

Epsilon-Aminocaproic Acid has been shown to increase serum potassium to clinically dangerous levels.

References

1. Perazella MA, Biswas P. Acute hyperkalemia associated with intravenous Epsilon-Aminocaproic Acid therapy. Am J Kidney Dis. 1999;33:782–5.
2. Nzerue CM, Falana B. Refractory hyperkalaemia associated with use of Epsilon-Aminocaproic Acid during coronary bypass in a dialysis patient. Nephrol Dial Transplant. 2002;17:1150–1.

Chapter 6
Case 6: An Adjuvant to the Cuff-Leak Test

You have just finished a long laparoscopic nephrectomy in a 50-year-old woman (5 ft 6 in. and 95 kg). She is the donor to her brother. The operation has lasted 7 h. Since she has been in Trendelenburg position for most of that time, her face and neck are very swollen. You are reluctant to remove the endotracheal tube (ETT) at the end of the surgery, although the surgeon sees no problem. You perform a leak test. This is traditionally done by auscultating the presence of breath sounds after deflating the cuff and occluding the ETT. You have difficulty hearing if an audible leak is present at the mouth [1]. You attempt the cuff-leak volume test (difference between inspiratory tidal volume and expiratory tidal volume while the cuff is deflated). This has been suggested to quantitatively predict postextubation outcomes [2]. However, you are not convinced that this patient's trachea can be safely extubated.

Question

Can you think of any other methods to ascertain if ETT can safely be removed?

J.G. Brock-Utne, *Case Studies of Near Misses in Clinical Anesthesia*,
DOI 10.1007/978-1-4419-1179-7_6,

Solution

You can ascertain the presence of end-tidal CO_2 by disconnecting the carbon dioxide/anesthetic agent sampling tube from the patient's breathing system. Then you can use the sampling tube to "sniff" the oral cavity to ascertain the presence of end-tidal carbon dioxide [3]. A similar "sniffing technique" using the sampling tube has been previously described to detect leaks in external vaporizers [4].

Measuring carbon dioxide at the mouth or inside the mouth may prove to be an adjunct to the leak test. If the leak tests and the "sniff" test are equivocal, than a gum elastic bougie or Aintree catheter (Cook Incorporated, Bloomington, IN) should be left in the trachea for rapid reintubation without the need for direct laryngoscopy [5]. If the original ETT had been a number 6 ETT or smaller, I would not have contemplated removing the ETT from the patient, but take her to the ICU for post-operative ventilation. It the surgeon then wants to extubate the patient in the ICU, then he will carry all responsibility.

Recommendation

Remember the "sniff technique" as an adjuvant to the cuff-leak test.

References

1. Potgieter PD, Hammond JM. "Cuff" test for safe extubation following laryngeal edema. Crit Care Med. 1988;16:818.
2. Miller RL, Cole RP. Association between reduced cuff leak volume and postextubation stridor. Chest. 1996;110:1035–40.
3. Eng MR, Wu TT, Brock-Utne JG. An adjuvant of the cuff leak test. Anaesthesia. 2009;64:452.
4. Bolton P, Brock-Utne JG, Zumaran AA, Cummings J, Armstrong D. A simple method to identify an external vaporizer leak (the "sniff" method). Anesth Analg. 2005;101:606–7.
5. Robles B, Hester J, Brock-Utne JG. Remember the gum-elastic bougie at extubation. J Clin Anesth. 1993;5:329–31.

Chapter 7
Case 7: *Acinetobacter baumannii* Outbreak in an ICU – Can Our Equipment Be at Fault?

An outbreak of a multidrug-resistant *Acinetobacter baumannii* has occurred in your hospital ICU. One small child has died and five other patients are on ventilator support. Hygienic measures are intensified. This includes instructing the healthcare workers to strictly adhere to hand hygiene between and during bronchial washing, flushing gastric tubes, caring for wounds, and washing of patients. Supplies of utility goods at the patients' bedside are kept to a minimum. The rooms are cleaned more frequently, with particular attention paid to areas where dust is likely to gather.

After this outbreak, the surgical ICU is closed and cleaned extensively. No contamination is found in any of the ICU equipment, like respirators. Shortly after the ICU opens again, the outbreak strain is once more isolated from patients. A second investigation into possible causes of this contamination is started. Since most of the patients come from the operating room, an extensive examination of all the rooms and equipment is commenced. This includes ventilators, autoclave, cupboards, chairs, C-arms, monitors, keyboards and computers, air conditioner inlet and outlets, infusion equipment, microscopes, anesthesia machines including suction, operating table, and random samples from the floor, walls, and ceilings. All come back negative, with the exception of some respiratory ventilators and some continuous veno-venous hemofiltration machines. However, there is one item which later turns out to be positive which was not tested before. This is because during the testing it has been kept in the anesthesia technician's work and equipment room.

Question

What was this equipment?

J.G. Brock-Utne, *Case Studies of Near Misses in Clinical Anesthesia*,
DOI 10.1007/978-1-4419-1179-7_7,

Solution

Bair Hugger (Augustine Medical Inc., Eden Prairie, MN) was the culprit. Removing dust from the machines and replacing all dust filters, including the ones in the Bair Hugger (BH), brought an end to the outbreaks [1]. Another study has also warned that the BH may be a risk factor for infection [2].

We published a study in 2009 [3] which is summarized here. Under sterile conditions, cotton swabs were taken from the distal end of BH tubing and the filter of the BH housed in 29 operating rooms. All swabs were inoculated onto Petri dishes. Petri dishes were also exposed to ambient air from the 29 operating rooms. The study was done at the time when the BH filters were recommended to be changed (after 6 months or more than 500 h of usage). The old filters were discarded and replaced. Three months later, the above study was repeated. In the initial study, 8 out of 29 ORs had pathological growth. The distal ends of the Bair Huggers were positive for growth in 12 out of 29. Three BH filters were positive. Three months later, a repeat study of the 8 positive ORs, 12 distal ends, and the 3 BHs showed no growth. The importance of changing the Bair Hugger filters was confirmed. However, the optimum timing as to when the filters should be changed is not clear. More studies are obviously needed. As an added safety feature, it has been recommended that an additional microbial filter be fitted to the distal end of the BH hose [4].

Recommendation

Don't forget to change the BH filter regularly. Failure to do so can prove disastrous for patients.

References

1. Bernards AT, Harinch HIJ, Dijkshoorn L, et al. Persistent *Acinetobacter baumannii*? Look inside your medical equipment. Infect Control Hosp Epidemiol. 2004;25:1002–4.
2. Huagn JKC, Shah EF, Vinokumar N, et al. The Bair Hugger patient warming system in prolonged vascular surgery: an infection risk? Crit Care. 2003;7:13–6.
3. Gjolai MP, Ahlbrand S, Yamout IM, Armstrong D, Brock-Utne JG. Don't forget to change the Bair Hugger filter. Anesthesiology. 2009, A1168.
4. Avidan MS, Jones N, Khoosal M, Lundgren C, Morrell DF. Convection warmers – not just hot air. Anaesthesia. 1997;52:1073–6.

Chapter 8
Case 8: A Complication with the Use of the Intubating Fiberscope

A 40-year-old man (65 kg, 5 ft 8 in.) is scheduled for a transoral decompression and posterior fixation of an atlanto-axial dislocation. He is otherwise healthy and has no lung disease.

An awake fiberoptic intubation is planned. Adequate oral analgesia with lidocaine 4% and cocaine 4% using an atomizer (Mucosal Atomizer Devicc, Wolfe Tory Medical, Salt Lake City, UT) is achieved. The patient is given midazolam, glycopyrrolate, and meperidine for sedation. The endotracheal tube (ETT) is loaded on the fiberscope and a long catheter is inserted through the forceps port of the fiberscope. This catheter is used to administer local anesthesia on the vocal cords should that be needed. Excellent local anesthesia and sedation is achieved, without the use of the long catheter. The fiberscope and the ETT are easily inserted into the trachea. The cuff on the ETT is blown up. The patient remains comfortable and shows little sign of distress with the ETT in the trachea. Unfortunately, the fiberscope is not easily removed from the ETT, but comes out using some force. However, after the removal of the fiberscope you notice that the long catheter is still inside the ETT. An attempt is made to pull out the long catheter, but it won't shift even with moderate force. The patient is still comfortable and is breathing spontaneously. He is oblivious of your problem.

Questions

Now what will you do? Cut the catheter?

J.G. Brock-Utne, *Case Studies of Near Misses in Clinical Anesthesia*,
DOI 10.1007/978-1-4419-1179-7_8, © Springer Science+Business Media, LLC 2011

Solutions

The first thing to do is to reinsert the fiberscope over the catheter into the ETT to try and elucidate the problem. You now see that the catheter has gone beyond the ETT and is lying in the trachea. You cannot see the tip. The catheter can still not be removed. You wonder if the catheter has migrated up between the ETT and the trachea and is stuck there by the ETT's cuff that is now blown up. You let the cuff down and the catheter comes out easily.

If the above maneuver had not worked then the only thing to do is to remove the ETT, fiberscope, and catheter in one and reintubate.

It has been recommended [1] that to minimize this kind of problem with the injection catheter it should be fixed with adhesive tape at the inlet of the forceps port. In this way, it can't protrude from the tip of the fiberscope.

Another complication with fiberscope intubation has been described [2]. In this case, the tip of fiberscope is placed inadvertently out of the Murphy's eye instead of the distal end of the ETT. This occurs if you do not pay attention.

Recommendation

A long catheter, inserted through the fiberscope for injection of local anesthetic onto the vocal cords, can become a problem. When using such a catheter, it is advisable to fix the catheter with tape, as it emerges from the fiberscope.

References

1. Prakash PS, Pandia MP. A complication associated with the use of a drug injection catheter through a fiberscope. Anesthesiology. 2008;108:173.
2. Nichols KP, Zornow HM. A potential complication of fiberoptic intubation. Anesthesiology. 1989;70:562–3.

Chapter 9
Case 9: Interscalene Block a Concern in Cardiac Patients?

An 83-year-old man (81 kg and 172 cm) is scheduled for an elective right shoulder arthroscopy with rotator cuff tear repair. His past medical history is significant for coronary artery disease. He has had two prior coronary artery bypass surgeries, the latest 12 years ago. Hypertension and hyperlipidemia are well controlled. On questioning, he denies any symptoms of chest pain or shortness of breath with exertion. EKG shows normal sinus rhythm and a right bundle branch block. A stress echocardiogram performed 2 weeks ago showed a normal ejection fraction with no signs of ventricular wall motion abnormalities. His oxygen saturation is 97% and his vital signs are normal. A chest X-ray was not ordered as his chest exam is normal except for decreased air entry at the base of the right lung.

An interscalene block is performed under sedation. A total of 40 mL of 0.5% ropivacaine with 1:400,000 epinephrine is injected with no complication. Complete sensory and motor block of the right shoulder are achieved within 15 min after the injection. Subsequently, general anesthesia is induced in a routine manner and an endotracheal intubation performed uneventfully. At the end of a 2-h surgery, the patient wakes up and his ETT is removed in the OR. He is taken to the recovery, awake, pain free, and with vital signs stable.

Shortly after arriving in the recovery area, the patient begins to complain of vague chest pain and shortness of breath. Auscultation of the chest reveals decreased breath sounds on the right side from the base to halfway up his chest. This is very different from the preoperative exam. There are no wheezes, rales, or rhonchi. A 12-lead EKG reveals no new ST segment changes compared with previous EKGs. Serial cardiac enzymes are negative.

J.G. Brock-Utne, *Case Studies of Near Misses in Clinical Anesthesia*,
DOI 10.1007/978-1-4419-1179-7_9,

The chest X-ray reveals interposition of a portion of the colon between the liver and right hemidiaphragm. The right hemidiaphragm is markedly elevated but no evidence of a pneumothorax.

Questions

What is the diagnosis? What happened?

Solution

The interposition of the colon between the liver and right hemidiaphragm is called the Chilaiditi's sign. This is a complication of open cardiac surgery. Furthermore, phrenic nerve injury following cardiac surgery has a variable incidence of 10–85% depending on the method of detection and patient population [1]. Urmey et al. [2] found phrenic nerve block to occur in 100% of interscalene block. However, patients with interscalene blocks do not experience a decrease in many pulmonary function variables including FVC and FEV1 [3]. Fujimura et al. [4] showed a decrease in PaO_2 after interscalene block in healthy volunteers most likely secondary to increased ventilation and perfusion mismatches. However, both studies (2 and 4) were done in healthy volunteers or ASA class 1 and 2. Studies have shown that reducing local anesthetic volume and applying digital pressure above the injection site do not reduce the rate of diaphragmatic and respiratory dysfunction [5, 6].

Several case reports have demonstrated postoperative dyspnea after interscalene block in patients with obesity, previous pulmonary disease, and recent cardiac surgery [7–9].

It is possible that this patient may have had some decreased respiratory reserve due to diaphragmatic dysfunction, even though the cardiac surgery was 12 years ago. Most cardiac patients fully recover phrenic nerve function within a year; however, a significant minority does not [1].

Messina et al. [10] has reported a case of respiratory distress in a patient with Chilaiditi's syndrome secondary to external compression of bronchial structures by the ectopically located colon. In the above patient the mass effect of the ectopically located colon on the diaphragm reduced the FRC even more. This helps explain why he developed dyspnea after hemidiaphragm paralysis. We have seen such a case whose dyspnea improved over hours [11]. He was discharged from the hospital the next day without any respiratory symptoms and his right hemidiaphragm elevation dramatically reduced.

Recommendation

When you contemplate an interscalene block in a patient who has had open cardiac surgery, it is imperative to have a preoperative chest X-ray. Should the Chilaiditi's syndrome be present, an interscalene block may not be advisable.

References

1. Dimopoulou I, Dagnou M, Dafni U, Karakatsani A, Khoury M, Geroulanus S, et al. Phrenic nerve dysfunction after cardiac operations: electrophysiologic evaluation of risk factors. Chest. 1998;113:8–14.

2. Urmey WF, Talts KH, Sharrock NE. One hundred percent incidence of hemidiaphragmatic paresis associated with interscalene brachial plexus anesthesia as diagnosed by ultrasonography. Anesth Analg. 1991;72:498–503.
3. Urmey WF, McDonald M. Hemidiaphragmatic paresis during interscalene brachial plexus block: effects on pulmonary function and chest wall mechanics. Anesth Analg. 1992;74:352–7.
4. Fujimura N, Namba H, Tsunoda K, Kawamata T, Taki K, Igarasi M, et al. Effect of hemidiaphragmatic paresis caused by interscalene brachial plexus block on breathing pattern, chest wall mechanics and arterial blood gases. Anesth Analg. 1995;81:962–6.
5. Urmey WF, Grossi P, Sharrock NE, Stanton J, Gloeggler PJ. Digital pressure during interscalene block is clinically ineffective in preventing anesthetic spread to the cervical plexus. Anesth Analg. 1996;83:366–70.
6. Urmey WF, Gloeggler PJ. Pulmonary function changes during interscalene brachial plexus block: effects of decreasing local anesthetic injection volume. Reg Anesth. 1993;18:244–9.
7. Hashim MS, Shevde K. Dyspnea during interscalene block after recent coronary bypass surgery. Anesth Analg. 1999;89:55–6.
8. Rau RH, Chan YL, Chuang HI, Cheng CR, Wong KL, Wu KH, et al. Dyspnea resulting from phrenic nerve paralysis after interscalene brachial plexus block in an obese male – a case report. Acta Anaesthesiol Sin. 1997;35:113–8.
9. Koscielniak-Nielsen ZJ. Hemidiaphragmatic paresis after interscalene supplementation of insufficient axillary block with 3 ml of 2% mepivacaine. Acta Anaesthesiol Scand. 2000;44:1160–2.
10. Messina M. Paolucci E, Casoni G, Gurioli C and Poletti V. A case of severe dyspnea and an unusual bronchoscopy. The Chilaiditi Syndrome. Respiration. 2008;76:216–7.
11. Sun N, Singh VM, Nguyen J, Brock-Utne JG. Interscalene block in a patient with previous open cardiac surgery (Submitted for publication, 2011).

Chapter 10
Case 10: Epidural Analgesia for Labor – Watch Out

A 42-year-old female (85 kg 5 ft 8 in.) is requesting an epidural for labor pain. She is a para 3 and has had epidurals in the past without any problem. Previous medical history is noncontributory and she has had no surgeries. The epidural is inserted uneventfully. The patient is placed on a continuous epidural infusion of 0.2% ropivacaine at a rate of 8 mL/h with patient-controlled epidural analgesia (PCEA) bolus setting at 6 mL/30 min using an epidural pump (Painsmart IOD, model #360-1101, Curlin Medical, Huntington Beach, CA 92649). The pump is placed above her by about 10 in. (30 cm) and attached to an IV pole. This is usual procedure, so the staff does not have to bend down to change the settings. The patient delivers a healthy boy 2 h later. After the episiotomy repair, the pump is turned off. Thirty minutes later no motor block is present. The patient received a total of approximately 40 mL of ropivacaine. She is very satisfied with your epidural and thanks you profusely. As she has consented for a tubal ligation, the epidural catheter is left in situ but as, mentioned, the pump is turned off.

However, 2 h later you are called back urgently. The patient is now complaining of bilateral complete motor block and a sensory level at T-8. The patient and her husband are looking at you anxiously.

You establish that the epidural pump is turned off. But you notice that the 60 mL syringe attached to the pump is empty. There should have been at least 20 mL left. You feel the bottom of the pump and look at the floor under the pump but see no evidence of any leak from the pump.

Questions

What will you do? What do you think has happened?

J.G. Brock-Utne, *Case Studies of Near Misses in Clinical Anesthesia*,
DOI 10.1007/978-1-4419-1179-7_10, © Springer Science+Business Media, LLC 2011

Solution

You reassure her that she will be fine.

You tell the patient that it looks like the epidural pump may be at fault. Even though the pump is turned off, it may still have infused the local anesthetic. You now disconnect the epidural infusion system from the epidural catheter and remove the epidural catheter intact from the patient. The patient is put on continuous monitoring and reassured. After 6–8 h, the patient has made a full recovery. In the meantime, you have confirmed your suspicion that the pump continued to delivered fluid after being shut off (Omid Khodadadi, 2009, personal communication). On examining the pump, you discover that the compressible portion of the epidural infusion set is seated on a conveyor belt. The belt has propulsive ridges on its surface. When the pump is turned off, these ridges occlude the softer portion of the tubing, thus shutting off flow. If the ridges fail to shut off the flow, the syringe can still empty because of the hydrostatic pressure. You establish that the higher the syringe is above the patient's epidural site, the more the flow. It would seem that the cause of the problem was normal wear and tear and/or damage caused by careless handling. Most of the time, it is no way of knowing when an infusion pump will malfunction [1].

Recommendation

Remember, when you order an epidural pump to be turned off, you should always disconnect the infusion system from the epidural catheter.

Reference

1. Grover ER, Heath ML. Patient-controlled analgesia. A serious incident. Anaesthesia. 1992;47:402–4.

Chapter 11
Case 11: Past History of Esophagectomy – Any Concern?

A 55-year-old man (68 kg, height 5 ft 10 in.) is scheduled for extensive dental work under general anesthesia. Two months before, he underwent successfully an Ivor Lewis midesophagus esophagectomy. He can now take multiple small meals and has gained weight. He is otherwise healthy. He has not had anything to eat or drink for 10 h.

Questions

What will be your anesthesia induction? Would you do a rapid sequence induction with cricoid pressure? If so, why?

J.G. Brock-Utne, *Case Studies of Near Misses in Clinical Anesthesia*,
DOI 10.1007/978-1-4419-1179-7_11, © Springer Science+Business Media, LLC 2011

Solutions

There are few reports in the literature that describe the risk of gastric aspiration following induction of general anesthesia in patient with a previous history of esophagectomy [1–3]. These reports should be taken seriously, as a very high proportion of these cases aspirate gastric content into the patient's lungs during induction of general anesthesia [1].

Esophagectomy results in excision of the lower esophageal sphincter (LES) and loss of vagal innervations of the stomach. Also the denervated stomach requires a pyloroplasty to prevent gastric outlet obstruction. Remember also that the flaccid stomach is situated in the thorax and is drained only by gravity.

There are various options for management of these cases and they include the following:

1. Placements of a soft oral/nasal tube prior to induction do decompress the stomach. However, the surgeon will have to agree that it is safe to place such a tube in the repaired esophagus. You do not want to cause an anastomotic disruption of the esophagus.
2. An awake fiberoptic induction with the patient in a sitting-up position [4].

The use of cricoid pressure in these cases is questionable as it is in patients with a normal esophagus [5, 6]. The use of cricoid pressure has not been shown to decrease the aspiration risk [5–7]. This may be related to the fact that cricoid pressure does not compress the cervical esophagus all the time [8]. Furthermore, cervical esophageal anastomosis may be lateral rather than posterior to the cricoids cartilage [1].

Since the LES is gone, the use of metoclopramide to increase LES tone serves no purpose. However, preoperative antacid should be given and may be beneficial.

Recommendation

In these cases, an awake fiberoptic induction, with the patient in the sitting position, may be the best option (See more discussion in case 20).

References

1. De Souza DG, Gaugen CL. Aspiration risk after esophagectomy. Anesth Analg. 2009; 109:1352.
2. Black DR, Thangathurai D, Senthikumar N, Roffey P, Mikhail M. High risk of aspiration and difficult intubation in postesophagecotmy patients. Acta Anaesthesiol Scand. 1999;43:687.
3. Jankovic ZB, Miklosavljevic S, Stamenkovic D, Stojakov D, Sabjljak P, Pesko P. High risk of aspiration and difficult intubation in post-esophagectomy patients. Acta Anaesthesiol Scand. 2000;44:899–900.

4. Brock-Utne JG, Jaffe RA. Endotrachela intubation with the patient in a sitting position. Br J Anaesth. 1991;67:225–6.
5. Ng A, Smith G. Gastroesphageal reflux and aspiration of gastric contents in anesthetic practice. Anesth Analg. 2001;93:494–513.
6. Brock-Utne JG. Is cricoid pressure necessary? Paediatr Anaesth. 2002;12:1–4.
7. Brimacombe JR, Berry AM. Cricoid pressure. Can J Anaesth. 1997;44:414–25.
8. Smith KJ, Dobranowski J, Yip G, Dauphin A, CHoi PT. Cricoid pressure displaces the esophagus: an observational study using magnetic resonance imaging. Anesthesiology. 2003;99:60–4.

Chapter 12
Case 12: A Case of Myasthenia Gravis

Today you are assigned to anesthetize a 52-year-old man with myasthenia gravis (MG) for a coiling of his cerebral aneurysm. Myasthenia gravis was diagnosed 9 months ago. The cerebral aneurysm is an incidental finding. You meet the patient in the preoperative holding area. He weighs 68 kg and is 5 ft 9 in. tall. He tells you that, a week ago, his neurologist increased his pyridostigmine dose. He thinks he is less weak now than he was a week ago. But he is not sure when questioned. He has no ptosis and/or diplopia. You do not detect any speech or swallowing difficulties. You review the lung functions test which was taken 3 weeks ago. The tests were done on the old medication dosing. All the values are as expected reduced, but they are acceptable to you. He is otherwise healthy. When you asked him to cough, you conclude he has a rather weak cough. The case is scheduled for 3 h.

Questions

1. Are you concerned? If so why?
2. Are there any other questions that you would like to ask him? If so what?
3. What are the three variables that you must anticipate in the management of all MG patients coming for surgery?

J.G. Brock-Utne, *Case Studies of Near Misses in Clinical Anesthesia*,
DOI 10.1007/978-1-4419-1179-7_12, © Springer Science+Business Media, LLC 2011

Solutions

1. A weak cough is very serious concern. I canceled the above patient based on the information above. I referred him back to his neurologist and to come back when he was on an optimum pyridostigmine dose. He should also be rescheduled for new pulmonary function tests (on the present medication dose). If the patient cannot cough postoperatively, then he may be at risk for pneumonia and need of prolonged postoperative ventilation with pulmonary toilet. If he has to be ventilated postoperatively, then getting him safely off the ventilator can prove to be a very difficult.
2. Even though the patient recently had his medication changed and states that he feels fine, you need to enquire about any possible evidence of excess pyridostigmine for example diarrhea. This is a most important question as new onset of diarrhea could indicate that he is getting too much treatment. The weakness in these patients, caused by an excess drug dose, can come on insidiously. Remember that weakness due to excessive drug treatment can be confused with weakness due to the myasthenia. Cholinergic crises can develop and the patient may require ventilation. In the above mentioned patient's case, the neurologist called back a week later and agreed with my assessment that the patient was getting too much pyridostigmine.
3. What are the three variables when dealing with a patient with myasthenia gravis coming for general anesthesia?
   (a) The preoperative medication. Is it optimum?
   (b) The muscle weakness produced by disease. Respiratory and bulbar weakness may predispose the patient to aspiration postoperatively. Can he hold his head up off the pillow? Can he cough adequately? Lung function tests are essential and they must be performed on the patient's current medication. Preoperatively, you can do the Snyder Match test. This consists of the patient holding a burning match at 8–10 in. (20–30 cm) and without pursing his/her lips blows out the candle.
   (c) The surgeon's need for muscle relaxation. If the surgeon can do without, then don't use any. In cerebral coiling, the patient requires full muscle relaxation. This is a one of the surgical procedures where moving during the procedure can be life threatening for the patient. If he does, it can prove to be an instant disaster for the patient.

Recommendation

Adequate coughing, optimum medication, and the need for muscle relaxation are questions that must be answered satisfactorily prior to anesthetizing a patient with MG.

Chapter 13
Case 13: Where Are My Teeth?

A 40-year-old man is scheduled for left ureteroscopic laser lithotripsy for nephrolithiasis. He is 90 kg and 5 ft 11 in. tall. His previous medical history is noncontributory. He had an uneventful hernia repair under general anesthesia 4 years ago. The anesthesia record mentioned no problem with endotracheal intubation. Examination of his airway reveals a maxillary anterior fixed partial denture. He informs you that they are "permanent." He has had the bridge for 17 years and never caused any problems. After a routine induction of anesthesia, the patient is easily mask ventilated. A grade-1 view of the larynx is achieved with an atraumatic direct laryngoscope and an endotracheal tube (ETT) placed easily into the trachea. The rest of the anesthesia is uneventful. At the end of the surgery, the patient's ETT is removed without any problems. He is transported to the postoperative care unit. Here, he experiences a bout of coughing. Upon becoming more alert, he says: "Where are my teeth?"

You examine him and find that indeed the front incisors where his fixed partial denture has been are now missing. He informs you that this has never happened before and he does not think he has swallowed them.

Question

The patient is very unhappy. What will you do now?

J.G. Brock-Utne, *Case Studies of Near Misses in Clinical Anesthesia*,
DOI 10.1007/978-1-4419-1179-7_13,

Solution

We have previously described such a case [1].

Since he was sure he had not swallowed the teeth, we searched the operating room, the hallways, and the recovery room thoroughly, but to no avail. An abdominal X-ray revealed a radio-opaque foreign body consistent in shape with the missing fixed particle denture overlying the stomach. A gastroenterologist was consulted while the patient was in the recovery room. An emergent upper endoscopy was done within 2 h of his arrival in the recovery room. However, the bridge was not visualized endoscopically. Repeat X-rays revealed that the bridge had passed into the small intestine. The patient was observed for a total of 3.5 h in the recovery room. Since he did not complain of any abdominal pain, nausea, or exhibited fever or hematomesis, he was discharged to the ward and the next day to home. On postoperative day 3, the bridge was passed into the stool without any problems.

Recommendation

Be observant about so-called "permanent teeth."

Reference

1. Lau G, Kulkarni V, Roberts GK, Brock-Utne JG. "Where are my teeth?" A case of unnoticed ingestion of a dislodged fixed partial denture. Anesth Analg. 2009;109:836–8.

Chapter 14
Case 14: An Unusual Capnograph Tracing

A 54-year-old (160 cm and 90 kg) woman is scheduled for right front temporal craniotomy for superficial temporal artery to middle cerebral artery bypass. Her past history was significant for bilateral Moyamoya disease, atrial aneurysm, obstructive sleep apnea, hypertension, and hyperlipidemia. You perform a preoperative check of the anesthetic machine (Apollo, Drager Medical, Telford, PA) including a leak test. No abnormalities are found.

During preoxygenation, you observe what appears to be a normal capnograph tracing. The patient is anesthetized in a routine manner with muscle relaxation, and the trachea is intubated with an endotracheal tube (ETT). Correct position of the ETT is confirmed with bilateral breath sounds and end-tidal CO_2 seen on the capnograph. The ETT is secured at 23 cm at the lip. You now notice an abnormal capnographic waveform with single hump midplateau (Fig. 14.1). The vital signs were end-tidal CO_2=36 mmHg, tidal volume 500 mL, peak inspiratory pressure=30 cm H_2O, respiratory rate=10, and the inspiratory to expiratory ratio=1:4. You change out the sampling system, as you think there is a leak. However, there is no change in the waveform with the new sampling system.

J.G. Brock-Utne, *Case Studies of Near Misses in Clinical Anesthesia*,
DOI 10.1007/978-1-4419-1179-7_14,

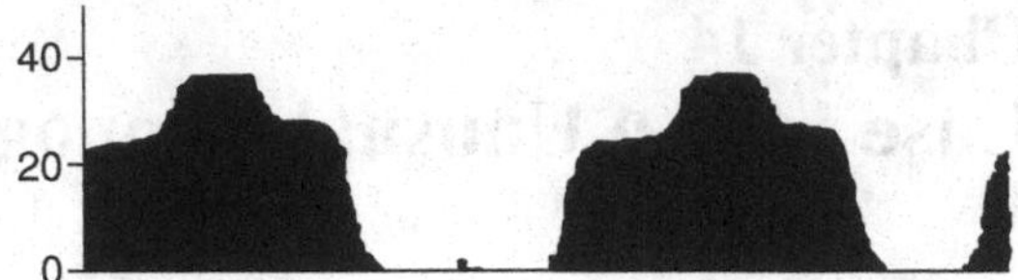

Fig. 14.1 Abnormal capnographic waveform with single hump midplateau. Reprinted, with permission, from Jaffe et al. [1]

Question

What can be the cause of this abnormal waveform?

Solution

The cause of this midplateau hump was due to a longer than normal sample line combined with a cracked water trap (Apollo Drager Medical, Telford, PA). We have previously published this finding and called it the Dromedary sign [1]. We believe the reason for this is an increased dyssynchrony between the positive pressure phase of mechanical ventilation and the arrival of the end-tidal gas, sampled at the elbow connector, at the gas analyzer. During expiration, negative pressure at the crack in the water trap allowed room air to dilute the sample. This leads to a decrease in end-tidal CO_2 concentration, seen as the first plateau. At the initiation of positive pressure by the ventilator, the negative pressure at the cracked water trap is reversed as the piston exerts positive pressure (peak inspiratory pressure), represented by the higher plateau hump. The higher plateau most accurately represents end-tidal CO_2 as sample dilution is eliminated. The third plateau is due to the increased sample line volume. This increases the dead space and therefore the time between expiration and the arrival of end-tidal CO_2 to the analyzer.

Therefore, the transit time delay caused by the additional dead space in the sample line combined with a cracked water trap resulted in the appearance of the Dromedary sign.

A biphasic, dual plateau waveform has been described [2] (Fig. 14.2). The cause of this abnormal wave form is due to room air being drawn into the sample line before it enters the analyzer. This is often caused by a leak or a loose connection anywhere between the elbow connector and the gas analyzer. During expiration, the room air enters the sample line because of the negative pressure caused by the sampling pump's suction. The entrained air dilutes the expiratory CO_2 in the sample. However, with the onset of positive pressure mechanical ventilation, the pressure gradient across the leak reverses. The leak is now outward, thereby eliminating the dilution effect. The result is a late expiratory plateau prior to the normal down slope of the capnograph waveform. Since CO_2 was not used during the preoperative machine check, the problem was not discovered.

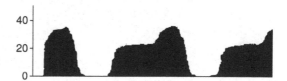

Fig. 14.2 Biphasic, dual plateau waveform. Reprinted, with permission, from Jaffe et al. [1]

Recommendation

This case illustrates the need to be able to deduce the cause of an abnormal capnography tracing. Understanding how the capnography works is essential for safe anesthesia practice.

References

1. Jaffe RA, Talavera JA, Hah JM, Brock-Utne JG. The Dromedary sign – an unusual capnograph tracing. Anesthesiology. 2008;109:49–50.
2. Body SC, Taylor K, Phillip J. Dual-plateau capnogram caused by cracked sample filter. Anesth Analg. 2000;90:233–4.

Chapter 15
Case 15: A VP Shunt

A 76-year-old female is scheduled for an emergency VP shunt. Two weeks prior, she had a craniotomy for a cerebral aneurysm. She is now obtunded and responds only to painful stimuli. Her vital signs are stable and she is breathing spontaneously. She has a naso-gastric feeding tube in situ. The last feed was 6 h ago. She weighs 68 kg and is 5 ft 8 in. tall. The surgeon tells you that he wants the mean arterial pressure (MAP) to be 80 mmHg and that the surgery will be less than 1 h.

Questions

1. Would you remove the naso-gastric tube prior to induction?
2. Would you consider a preoperative arterial line?
3. Would you use muscle relaxation in this case?

J.G. Brock-Utne, *Case Studies of Near Misses in Clinical Anesthesia*,
DOI 10.1007/978-1-4419-1179-7_15,

Solutions

1. Removal of the naso-gastric tube is controversial [1, 2]. I would think it is worthwhile as the tube makes both the upper and lower esophageal sphincters incompetent. Whatever you decide, it is important to verify from the nurses notes that when the last naso-gastric feed was done. Looking at the nurses records is essential in this case. Also you should attempt to suck out any stomach content, prior to the anesthetic induction. An antacid injected through the naso-gastric tube is recommended.
2. An arterial line should be inserted preoperatively to maintain the MAP at 80 mmHg. Vasopressors may have to be used to maintain the MAP at the desired level.
3. After preoxygenation, induction of anesthesia should be with an intravenous induction agent with or without the use of alfentanil 500–750 μg. Cricoid pressure should be performed and the endotracheal intubation should be without the use of muscle relaxation drugs. Maintenance should be with isoflurane in oxygen. When the patient's respiration returns, the operation can begin. Should the end tidal CO_2 be elevated above desired levels, then assisted ventilation can be performed. However, the patient should keep breathing spontaneously.

Why is it important not to use muscle relaxation? After the surgery has started, it is most likely that any changes to the spontaneous respiration, rate, and rhythm can be attributed to the surgical procedure. Hence, respiration becomes a neurological monitor. Some anesthesiologist colleagues of mine use a LMA, instead of an ETT. This must be considered more risky, as the patient's head is most often turned 180° away from you and the anesthesia machine. If you select this option, the LMA you should consider is Dr. Brain's Supreme LMA (The Laryngeal Mask company Ltd. Le Rocher, Victoria, Mahe, Seychelles).

Recommendation

Remember in these cases, the respiration can be the most important neurological monitor.

References

1. Ng A, Smith G. Gastresophageal reflux and aspiration of gastric contents in anesthesia practice. Anesth Analg. 2001;93:494–513.
2. Brock-Utne JG. Gastresophageal reflux and aspiration of gastric contents in anesthesia practice. Anesth Analg. 2002;94:762.

Chapter 16
Case 16: Shoulder Surgery – Watch Out!

Today you are anesthetizing a 38 year old man (90 kg and 185 cm) for shoulder reconstruction. The patient is otherwise healthy and does not take any medication regularly. He has not had any surgery in the past. A surgeon, you have never worked with, is going to do the surgery. The patient is anesthetized in a routine manner with fentanyl, propofol, and rocuronium. The trachea is intubated using a #9 endotracheal tube (ETT). The ETT is secured at 22 cm. The patient receives positive-pressure ventilation. Anesthesia is maintained with sevoflurane in oxygen. The patient is placed in a beach chair position and his left arm is placed on a McConnell armholder (Greenville, TX 75401) and secured. You have not seen anyone use this armholder before. The surgery commences. Two hours later there is a sudden drop in systolic pressure to 60 mmHg, measured at the right ankle. The heart rate goes from 60 to 110 bpm and the end-tidal CO_2 decreases from 30 to 15 mmHg. The oxygen saturation decreases from 100 to 85%. The ventilator parameters all remain the same. You cannot see any obvious blood loss nor have you given any medications for over 1.5 h.

You diagnose iatrogenic venous air embolism and ask the surgeon to flood the field while you drop the head of the patient. The surgeon shouts: "Stop. Don't lower the head of the bed before I…."

Question

What is that the surgeon wants to do before you can place the patient in Trendelenburg?

J.G. Brock-Utne, *Case Studies of Near Misses in Clinical Anesthesia*,
DOI 10.1007/978-1-4419-1179-7_16, © Springer Science+Business Media, LLC 2011

Solution

It is very important to realize that the McConnell is attached to the sidebar of the operating room table. Since the patient's arm is on the McConnell armrest, it is locked in too. Hence, when you lower the beach chair you will dislocate the humeral head anteriorly and potentially cause serious damage to the bone and the surrounding structures.

This happened to me and luckily the surgeon managed to undo the McConnell quickly. The patient was quickly placed in Trendelenburg and the blood pressure and oxygenation improved within minutes. The patient made an uneventful recovery and was discharged home the next day.

The importance of not using N_2O in these cases should be stressed. Remember that N_2O moves into the air-filled body spaces 34 times faster than nitrogen can leave. This can lead to a dramatic increase in volume size.

If the Trendelenburg and flooding the field had not improved matters then other causes of acute intraoperative cardiovascular collapse should have been considered. In trauma cases these include: cardiac tamponade, fat embolism, hemolytic transfusion reactions, or tension pneumothorax. In elective case: myocardial infarction, anaphylaxis to medications, and acute hypovolemia are things you should consider.

Approximately, 9% of normal patients have a flow patent foramen ovale [1, 2]. Hence in those cases, venous air may pass from the right to the left atrium and from there into the systemic circulation. Thereby causing an air embolus, the worst complications involving paradoxical emboli are cerebral and myocardial infarction.

Recommendation

The message of this story is that you must understand the function and potential pitfalls of all the equipment that is used for patient care in the operating room, including the surgeons.

References

1. Jaffe RA, Pinto FJ, Schnittger I, Brock-Utne JG. Intraoperative ventilator-induced right to left intracardiac shunt. Anesthesiology. 1991;75:153–5.
2. Jaffe RA, Pinto FJ, Schnittger I, Siegel LC, Wranne B, Brock-Utne JG. Aspects of mechanical ventilation affecting interarterial shunt flow during general anesthesia. Anesth Analg. 1992;75:484–8.

Chapter 17
Case 17: An Ambulatory Surgical Patient with No Escort

Today you are in a "stand alone" ambulatory center. A 25 year old man is scheduled for a knee arthroscopy for a medial meniscus tear. You see the patient preoperatively, take a history, and examine him. You declare him a healthy ASA 1. He weighs 83 kg and is 5 ft 11 in. tall. The nurse tells you he has no escort. A friend who was to escort him home is now unavailable. You reaffirm the need for him to be safely transported home with an escort. The patient is however very keen to proceed and agrees to a have the procedure done under local anesthesia. The surgeon gives the patient an injection in the surgical site, 20 mL of lidocaine 1% and 20 mL bupivacaine 0.5%. Everything goes well until after an hour the patient becomes restless and agitated. You give him IV midazolam 2 mg, fentanyl 50 μg, and incremental doses of 50 mg of propofol. The total dose of propofol is 150 mg.

In the recovery room he is able to drink, eat, and walk within 1 h of the surgery. He also urinates and claims he is "fit as a fiddle." He wants to drive home in his car.

Questions

How would you handle this? Let him drive home or what?

J.G. Brock-Utne, *Case Studies of Near Misses in Clinical Anesthesia*,
DOI 10.1007/978-1-4419-1179-7_17,

Solutions

Never let a person like this drive home. Two malpractice cases have highlighted this problem [1]. Both cases had local anesthetic with sedation and were discharged without an escort after an ambulatory surgical procedure. While driving themselves home, they both had car accidents and sustained serious injuries. In fact, one even became a quadriplegic. Both cases went to court. In the first case, like the one mentioned here, the anesthesiologist was found guilty but the orthopedic surgeon was let off. In the other case, a preoperative nurse, on the surgeons order, gave lorazepam 1 mg for sedation. No other medication was given IV. A D/C was done purely under local anesthesia provided by the surgeon. No anesthesiologist was in attendance. The patient drove herself home but had an accident. After the car accident she sued the preoperative nurse and surgeon. Both were found to be negligent for allowing the patient to drive herself home after sedation. A second car was involved in this latter accident and the injured parties in the second car also sued and were compensated.

Discharge from an ambulatory surgical center without an escort is contrary to the guidelines issued by the ASA, Canadian Anesthesiologists' Society, the Association of Anesthetists of Great Britain and the Australian Day Surgery council. The recommendations are supported by studies showing that psychomotor impairment and cognitive deficit are common in the recovery period [2–4]. These national guidelines make no distinction between sedation, regional anesthesia, and general anesthesia. Patient requires escorts to go home regardless of the type of anesthesia [1]. Studies [5, 6] have shown that most patients are not fully recovered and back to their normal functional status by the time the discharge criteria are met. Home readiness is not equal to street fitness [1].

As outlined previously, the major concern for patients without escort is that they will drive home after ambulatory surgery [1]. The above societies, with the exception of ASA recommend patients not drive for 24 h. Chung et al. [7] compared the driving performance (in a simulator) of patients who had their surgery performed under general anesthesia and compared these results to healthy volunteers. They showed that patients were impaired both pre- and postoperatively. The fact that patients were impaired preoperatively compared to controls must be due to the stress of the upcoming surgery [7]. This is important information.

One may ask what one would do if the patient had received only local anesthesia. In that case, most surgical centers will allow the patient to drive home. However, if the patient should receive sedation at any stage during his/her stay in the surgical center then the patient must not drive home. If there is no escort, then you order a taxi for transport. If the patient does not have money for a taxi – you pay. You do not want the money back but do remember to get a receipt. Paying for a taxi could prove safer and cheaper. However, it is imperative that you or a hospital staff makes sure the patient takes the taxi. Compliance can be an issue [8, 9].

Recommendation

It is not recommended to discharge a patient from an ambulatory surgical center without an escort to drive them home. This should be done irrespective if the patient had a general anesthetic, monitored care with or without sedation, or just regional anesthesia without sedation [1].

References

1. Chung F, Assmann N. Car accidents after ambulatory surgery in patients without an escort. Anesth Analg. 2008;106:817–20.
2. Grant SA, Murdoch J, Millar K, Kenny GNC. Blood propofol concentration and psychomotor effects on driving skills. Br J Anaesth. 2000;85:396–400.
3. Chung F, Seyone C, Dyck B, Chung A, Ong D, Taylor A, et al. Age related cognitive recovery after anesthesia. Anesth Analg. 1990;71:217–24.
4. Ward B, Imarengiaye C, Peirovy J, Chung F. Cognitive function is minimally impaired after ambulatory surgery. Can J Anaesth. 2005;52:1017–21.
5. Thapar P, Zacny JP, Thompson W, Apfelbaum JL. Using alcohol as a standard to assess the degree of impairment induced by sedative and analgesic drugs used in ambulatory surgery. Anesthesiology. 1995;82:53–9.
6. Lichtor JL, Alessi R, Lane BS. Sleep tendency as a measure of recovery after drugs used in ambulatory surgery. Anesthesiology. 2002;96:878–83.
7. Chung F, Kayumov L, Sinclair DR, Moller HJ, Shapiro CM. What is the driving performances of ambulatory surgical patients after general anesthesia? Anesthesiology. 2005;103:951–6.
8. Correa R, Menezes RB, Wong J, Yogendran S, Jenkins K, Chung F. Compliance with postoperative instruction: a telephone survey of 750 day surgery patients. Anaesthesia. 2001;56: 481–4.
9. Cheng CJC, Smith I, Watson BJ. A multicenter telephone survey of compliance with postoperative instructions. Anaesthesia. 2002;57:778–817.

Chapter 18
Case 18: A Complication During Laparoscopy

Today you are scheduled to anesthetize a 28-year-old female for removal of the right fallopian tube ectopic pregnancy. She is otherwise healthy and you give her an ASA 1 classification. She weighs 72 kg and is 5 ft 10 in. tall. A routine general anesthesia is induced and maintenance is with 1–2% sevoflurane and 70% nitrous oxide in oxygen. The surgeon places a transurethral bladder catheter and attaches it to a soft plastic collection bag. Pneumoperitoneum is created with insufflation of 100% carbon dioxide to a pressure of 16 mmHg. Fifteen minutes into the case you notice that the urinary collection bag has become very distended.

Questions

You diagnose a ruptured bladder and inform the surgeon. He is not happy and says to you: "How do you know?"

Is there any way you can quickly determine what the gas is and thereby convince the surgeon?

J.G. Brock-Utne, *Case Studies of Near Misses in Clinical Anesthesia*,
DOI 10.1007/978-1-4419-1179-7_18, © Springer Science+Business Media, LLC 2011

Solution

Rupture of the bladder during laparoscopic surgery is well described [1–3]. In these cases, the urinary collection bag is seen to suddenly distend dramatically due to CO_2 entering the bladder from the pneumoperitoneum.

To convince the surgeon that a urologic injury has occurred, you disconnect the CO_2/anesthetic agent sampling line from the capnograph at the elbow above the endotracheal tube. Thereafter, you attach a 20 gauge needle to the end of the sampling line. The needle is inserted into the top of the collection bag above the urine. If you are correct, then CO_2 will be seen on the capnograph. This should help to convince the surgeon "who never does anything wrong" that there is a problem [4]. To diagnose the presence of CO_2 in this way is similar to the described "sniff" method to diagnose a leaking vaporizer [5].

Recommendation

Rupture of the bladder during laparoscopic surgery is well documented. To convince a surgeon that the distention of the urinary bag is CO_2, is easily done using the capnograph.

References

1. Schanbacker PD, Rossi LJ, Salem MR, Joseph NJ. Detection of urinary bladder perforation during laparascopy by distension of the collection bag with carbon dioxide. Anesthesiology. 1994;80:680–1.
2. Classi RM, Sloan PA. Intraoperative detection of laparoscopic bladder injury. Can J Anaesth. 1995;42:415–6.
3. Sia-Kho E, Kelly RE. Urinary drainage bad distention: an indication of bladder injury during laparascopy. J Clin Anesth. 1992;4:346–7.
4. Valenta K, Brock-Utne JG. Confirmation of urinary bladder perforation during laparscopy. Remember the capnography (Submitted for publication 2011).
5. Bolton P, Brock-Utne JG, Sumaran AA, Armstrong D. A simple method to identify an external vaporizer leak (the "Sniff" method). Anesth Analg. 2005;101:606–7.

Chapter 19
Case 19: A Patient with Amyotrophic Lateral Sclerosis

Today you are assigned to anesthetize a patient with amyotrophic lateral sclerosis (ALS). He is 43 years old and weighs 65 kg and is 5 ft 10 in. tall. The patient is having diaphragmatic pacer (DPS) placed prophylactically. DPS is used to treat ventilator insufficiency in quadriplegic patients [1, 2]. The operation will be done laparoscopically. He is otherwise healthy with a forced vital capacity greater than 50% and a normal EKG. You premedicate him with 1 mg of midazolam and 10 mg of metoclopramide. In the operating room you place routine monitors and a remifentanil infusion of 0.05 mcg/kg/min is started. Anesthesia is induced with 150 mg of propofol. He is easily ventilated with 100% oxygen with 3% sevoflurane. No muscle relaxant is used at induction or at any time during the procedure. The trachea is sprayed with 160 mg of lidocaine (LTA 360 Kit, Hospira, Inc., Lake Forest, IL 60045) and a cuffed endotracheal tube (ETT) is placed. The correct placement of the ETT is confirmed with auscultation and end-tidal CO_2 waveform. The patient is then ventilated using an Apollo machine (Drager Medical, Telford, PA) with a tidal volume of 8–10 mg/kg and at a rate of 10–12 bpm. This Apollo machine can generate pressure volume (*P*/*V*) curves that can be visualized on the machine display. Anesthesia is maintained with the remifentanil infusion of 0.05 mcg/kg/min and a mixture of 30% oxygen, 70% nitrous oxide and sevoflurane titrated to achieve an end-tidal concentration of 1–1.5%. You are concerned that pneumoperitoneum cannot be adequately maintained since no muscle relaxation is used. However, this proves to be no problem [3].

The surgeon now places the pacing electrodes on each of the hemidiaphragm [1]. The ventilation by the Apollo machine is stopped and the ventilation maintained by the pacer only. The optimum placing of the DPS is established by measuring the maximal transdiaphragmatic pressure created by the electrodes. This is recorded by a transducer system outside the patient. You think this does not seem a very ideal way of establishing the optimum placement.

J.G. Brock-Utne, *Case Studies of Near Misses in Clinical Anesthesia*,
DOI 10.1007/978-1-4419-1179-7_19,

Question

Is there another method you can think of using in this case?

Solution

By comparing the *P*/*V* curve using the DPS and comparing that to the *P*/*V* loop generated with the Apollo ventilator, optimum pacing electrode placement can be achieved [3].

ALS is a relentlessly progressive neuromuscular disease of unknown origin. It affects both upper and lower motor neurons, causing weakness, hyperreflexia, and atrophy. It is important to realize that up to 80% of motor neurons are lost before the first clinical symptoms appear [4]. The disease affects more men than woman and life expectancy of ALS patients are 3–5 years after the diagnosis. Death usually occurs from respiratory complications.

Asai et al. [5] suggest that some of the ALS patients who die of Sudden Cardiac Arrest (SCA) have a prolonged QTC interval. In our study [3] of three ALS patients undergoing general anesthesia, one developed a temporary increase in QT interval but no adverse effects were seen. It may be prudent, when faced with these patients, to avoid drugs that can increase the QT interval like metoclopramide and ondansetron.

Recommendation

By comparing the *P*/*V* loop using the DPS with the *P*/*V* result generated by the anesthesia ventilator, optimum pacing electrode placement can be achieved. Also all ALS patients should have preoperative cardiac workup which should include an echocardiography.

References

1. Onders RP, Elmo KJ, Ignagni AR. Diaphragm pacing stimulation system for tetraplegia in individuals injured during childhood or adolescence. J Spinal Cord Med. 2007;30:S25–9.
2. Dimarco AF, Onders RP, Kowalski KE, Miller ME, Ferek S, Mortimer JT. Phrenic nerve pacing in a tetraplegic patient via intramuscular diaphragm electrode. Am J Respir Crit Care Med. 2002;166:1604–6.
3. Schmiesing CA, Lee J, Morton JM, Brock-Utne JG. Laparascopic diaphragmatic pacer placement – a potential new treatment for ALS patients: a brief description of the device and anesthestic issues. J Clin Anesth. 2010;22:549–52.
4. Mitusmuto H. The clinical features and prognosis in ALS. In: Mitsumoto H, Munsat T, editors. Amyotropic lateral sclerosis. A guide for patients and families. 2nd ed. New York: Demos; 2001. p. 27.
5. Asai H, Hirano M, Udaka F, Shimada K, Oda M, Kubori T, et al. Sympathetic disturbances increase risk of sudden cardiac arrest in sporadic ALS. J Neurol Sci. 2007;254:78–83.

Chapter 20
Case 20: Repair of a Thoracic Duct

A 72 year old man had undergone an uneventful transhiatal esophagectomy for Barrett's esophagitis. Ten days later he returns to the hospital with increasing shortness of breath. A large left pleural effusion is diagnosed. A chest tube is placed and creamy fluid was withdrawn. The chest tube continued to drain chylc and he is scheduled for repair of the thoracic duct. To identify the site of the injury to the duct, a 250 mL milk and heavy cream (50:50) mixture is ordered to be given 3 h prior to surgery. This is given, so that the surgeon can observe milky fluid dripping from the open thoracic duct and repair it.

On the day of surgery you establish that he is otherwise healthy. He still has an underwater drain which is working. There is decreased air entry in the left lung's mid and basal area. He confirms that he drank the heavy cream/milk mixture some time ago. You look at the nurse's notes and confirm that it has been given, but no time is given except to say this a.m.

You are obviously concerned about the possibility of pulmonary aspiration of the mixture and consider using a rapid sequence with cricoid pressure.

Questions

1. Is the latter any use in this case?
2. Is there anything else you may want to do prior to induction of general anesthesia?
3. What about the use of metoclopramide prior to induction of anesthesia to increase the lower esophageal sphincter?

DOI 10.1007/978-1-4419-1179-7_20,

Solutions

1. It is important to verify what has been done in the previous operation as to where the esophagus and/or stomach are. Cricoid pressure will be useless if there is no esophagus behind the cricoid ring but rather the stomach. Compressing the stomach will not prevent aspiration should it occur [1].
2. Always ascertain when the heavy cream/milk mixture was given. In a previous similar case [2], the patient aspirated on induction. This was not helped by the fact that, the mixture had only been given 30 min before induction of anesthesia. Administrating the milk/cream mixture via a jejunostomy tube may prove to be safer than per os [3].
3. Since there is a loss of sphincter tone following the initial surgery, the use of metoclopramide serves no purpose.

In the case mentioned earlier and the case referred to [2], the patient aspirated on induction of anesthesia. All maneuvers were done to alleviate the damage caused by the aspiration. This included tilting the head down, sucking out the pharynx, intubating the trachea with a double lumen tube, and sucking out the trachea and each bronchus vigorously prior to ventilation. Suction should be preferably done with a fiberoptic bronchoscopy.

The practice of oral administration of cream/milk mixture before surgery in these cases has been used since 1985. This case [2] would seem to be the only published report of aspiration of this material on induction of general anesthesia. Patients presenting for this surgery are probably at risk of aspiration for several reasons. After transhiatal esophagectomy, there is a loss of esophageal sphincter tone. The incidence of regurgitation is very high even without anesthesia. Orringer et al. [4] claim the regurgitation in these cases approaches 30%. In the patient described in [2], the interval between oral administration of cream/milk mixture and induction of anesthesia was only 30 min. Had one been aware of this, then a delay in the surgery for at least 3 h would have been a good idea. However, that may not have been enough. The safe interval to fast with this mixture in adults is unknown. For infants, at least a 3 h fast between the end of breast feeding to surgery is recommended [5]. An awake fiberoptic intubation may have been a better option in this case [6].

The patient survived the aspiration mainly due to the fact that the pH of the aspirate had a pH of 7 [7]. However, the clinical course following the aspiration was very similar to that reported after aspiration of clear liquids with a very low pH. This could mean that the pH is not so important with this mixture but rather the reaction of the lung to this aspirate.

Recommendation

Patients coming for surgery, with a history of a previous esophagectomy should be a concern to all anesthesiologists. This is especially true if a milk/cream mixture is given preoperatively.

References

1. Hoftman N. Cricoid pressure not protective in patients that have undergone esophagectomy. Anesth Analg. 2007;104:1303.
2. Brodsky JB, Brock-Utne AJ, Levi D, Ikonomidis JS, Whyte RI. Pulmonary aspiration of milk/cream mixture. Anesthesiology. 1999;91:1533–4.
3. Orringer MB, Bluett M, Deep GM. Aggressive treatment of chylothorax complicating transhiatal esophagectomy without thoracotomy. Surgery. 1988;104:720–6.
4. Orringer MB, Marshall B, Stirling MC. Transhiatal esophagectomy for benign and malignant disease. J Thorac Cardiovasc Surg. 1993;105:265–77.
5. Litman RS, Wu CL, Quinlivan JK. Gastric volume and pH in infants fed clear liquids and breast milk prior to surgery. Anesth Analg. 1994;79:482–5.
6. Brock-Utne JG, Jaffe RA. Endotracheal intubation with the patient in a sitting position. Br J Anaesth. 1991;67:225–6.
7. Raidoo DM, Rocke DA, Brock-Utne JG, Marszalek A, Engelbrecht HE. Critical volume for pulmonary acid aspiration. Reappraisal in a primate model. Br J Anaesth. 1990;65:248–50.

Chapter 21
Case 21: Occluded Reinforced (Armored) Endotracheal Tube

A 30 year old man is scheduled for a major ear nose and throat surgery. He has had a facial injury following a motor vehicle accident. The patient is otherwise healthy. You anesthetize him in a routine manner and secure the airway using a #8 armored endotracheal tube (ETT). The operation lasts for 10 h and the patient's face and neck is now very swollen. A tracheostomy had been planned to be donc at the end of the case but due to the swelling it was not done. The patient is instead taken to the ICU intubated with the armored tube for ventilation overnight. Since you are concerned about laryngeal edema you do not change the armored tube to a regular ETT over a tube changer.

The next morning the patient awakes from the sedation and bites vigorously on the armored ETT. Due to the nature of the ETT, the lumen becomes completely occluded and will not re-expand as the patient's mouth is opened. The patient cannot breath nor can the lungs be ventilated. The oxygen saturation falls to 80%. Cyanosis becomes evident. You can easily open his mouth.

Question

What will you do now?

J.G. Brock-Utne, *Case Studies of Near Misses in Clinical Anesthesia*,
DOI 10.1007/978-1-4419-1179-7_21, © Springer Science+Business Media, LLC 2011

Solution

A hemostat can easily manipulate the armored ETT into its near original shape by compressing the hemostat at 90° to the occlusion [1]. With the ETT near functioning again, you get the O_2 saturation up to 100%. If you then want/need to change the damaged ETT you can do that with tube changer or a gum-elastic-bougie [2]. If the tube changer or the bougie cannot be passed easily, cut the armored ETT below the obstruction and then pass the tube changer or the bougie.

Recommendation

Always have a bit block, not an oral airway or a soft airway in the mouth when an armored ETT is used. This is done to prevent occlusion [1] and/or biting the armored ETT in half [3, 4].

References

1. Vogel T, Brock-Utne JG. Solution to an occluded reinforced (armored) endotracheal tube. Am J Anesthesiol. 1997;2:58–61.
2. Robles B, Hester J, Brock-Utne JG. Remember the gum-elastic bougie at extubation. J Clin Anesth. 1993;5:329–31.
3. Kong CS. A small child can bite through an armored tracheal tube. Anaesthesia. 1995;50:263.
4. King H-K, Lewis K. Guedel oropharangeal airway does not prevent patient biting on the endotracheal tube. Anaesth Intensive Care. 1996;24(6):729–30.

Chapter 22
Case 22: A Difficult Nasogastric Tube Insertion

A 68 year old man is scheduled for an emergent exploratory laparotomy. Two weeks previously he had undergone a right hemicolectomy. He now presents with a 2 day history of severe abdominal pain, increasing abdomen distention, and the absence of passing wind and/or defecation. He is otherwise healthy. He is nil per os for 14 h. He weighs 68 kg and 5 ft 9 in. His other medical history is noncontributory. His airway is classified as Mallampati 1 and he is edentulous. Rapid sequence induction is uneventful and the endotracheal tube is inserted into the trachea and secured. The surgeons request a nasogastric (NG) tube. However, you find you are unable to pass the NG tube into the esophagus. You attempt to digitally manipulate the tip into the esophagus but to no avail. Visualizing the posterior oropharynx with either a different laryngoscopy blades and using a Magill forceps proves to be unsuccessful. You put the NG tube in ice making it stiffer for easier entry into the esophagus. However, it does not work and only creates an epistaxis.

Question

What will you now do to get the NG tube into the stomach?

J.G. Brock-Utne, *Case Studies of Near Misses in Clinical Anesthesia*,
DOI 10.1007/978-1-4419-1179-7_22,

Solution

The short GlideScope (Verathon, Bothell, WA 98011) provides a video view of the larynx during intubation. It is designed to help with securing the airway in difficult intubations. It is easy to master. Lifting up the epiglottis with the blade gives you a clear view of the laryngeal structures and the entrance to the esophagus. The NG tube can then be advanced manually into the esophagus [1].

The insertion of the NG tube in anesthetized, paralyzed, and intubated or unconscious patient has a 50% failure rate on the first attempt with the head in a neutral position [2, 3]. The most common site of stoppage of the NG tube is in the piriform sinuses and the arytenoid cartilage [4]. Once kinked, the NG tube is subsequently more likely to kink at the same place in the pharynx [5]. Common methods to facilitate the NG tube insertion include the use of a slit endotracheal tube, forward placement of the larynx and the use of various forceps, the use of an ureteral guidewire as a stylet, head flexion, using a gloved finger to steer the NG tube, and lateral neck pressure [3, 5–9]. The latter is my favorite as the later pressure occludes the piriform fossa and thereby prevents the NG tube to get stuck there.

Recommendation

Remember the GlideScope when you have difficulty placing an oral or nasogastric tube. It is a fact that placing these tubes can be one of the most challenging aspects of anesthesia practice. Any tips on how to make it easier is always welcome.

References

1. Hunter CW, Cohen S. A new use for the Glidescope. Anesth Analg. 2006;103:509.
2. Bong CL, Macachor JD, Hwang NC. Insertion of the nasogastric tube made easy. Anesthesiology. 2004;101:266.
3. Mahajan R, Gupta R. Another method to assist nasogastric tube insertion. Can J Anaesth. 2005;52:652–3.
4. Parris W. Reverse Sellick maneuver. Anesth Analg. 1989;68:423.
5. Appukuty J, Shroff PP. Nasogastric tube insertion using different techniques in anesthetized patients: a prospective, randomized study. Anesth Analg. 2009;109:832–5.
6. Ozer S, Benumof JL. Oro-nasogastric tube passage in intubated patients: fiberoptic description of where they go at the laryngeal level and how to make them enter the esophagus. Anesthesiology. 1999;91:137–43.
7. Flegar M, Ball A. Easier nasogastric tube insertion. Anaesthesia. 2004;59:197.
8. Sprague DH, Carter SR. An alternative method for nasogastirc tube insertion. Anesthesiology. 1980;53:436.
9. Campbell B. A novel method of nasogastric tube insertion. Anaesthesia. 1997;52:1234.

Chapter 23
Case 23: Antiphospholipid Antibody Syndrome – Any Concern for General Anesthesia?

A 42-year-old female (ASA 2) is scheduled for outpatient functional endoscopic sinus surgery. She has had no previous surgical procedures under anesthesia. She is otherwise healthy except for a history of hypertension, mild COPD, and antiphospholipid antibody syndrome. She is taken to the operating room and standard monitors are placed, including the oxygen saturation probe on her ring finger [1]. Routine general anesthesia proves uneventful. Her eyes are taped after she is asleep, but before the airway is secured with an endotracheal tube. The intraoperative course and extubation is uncomplicated. The tapes on her eyes are seen to have closed the eyelids throughout the operation. The eye tape is easily and atraumatically removed at the end of the surgery. The patient wakes up and is comfortable with no pain. The patient is taken to the recovery room. At no time was the patient seen rubbing her eyes, either on the way to the recovery or in the recovery room.

Twenty minutes later she complains of right eye discomfort. You examine the eye and conclude she has an injected right conjunctiva. There is no change in visual acuity.

Questions

What will you do? Why did this happen?

J.G. Brock-Utne, *Case Studies of Near Misses in Clinical Anesthesia*,
DOI 10.1007/978-1-4419-1179-7_23,

Solutions

Always call for an ophthalmology consult in these cases. In this case [2], a 1.5 cm linear longitudinal corneal abrasion was seen under fluorescein staining. The lesion was located along the inferior-media surface of the cornea. Based on the lesion's location and appearance the ophthalmologist concluded that the abrasion was most consistent with an excess dryness and not physical trauma. The patient was treated with antibiotic eye ointment, discharged home that evening, and made a complete recovery.

A review of the literature suggests a strong link between eye dryness and the development of corneal abrasions in patients with underlying autoimmune disease [2]. However, there is currently no literature that specifically documents this possible association. Since our case report [2], we have seen two additional patients with baseline chronic dry eyes undergoing general anesthesia for non-eye surgery. One of these patients specifically requested that we use ointment to prevent corneal abrasion. This request was based on a previous operative experience. The other patient had a know diagnosis of Sjogren syndrome and received saline intermittently throughout the case. None of these cases developed a corneal abrasion.

Ocular injuries, during general anesthesia for nonocular surgery, are still prevalent. The majority of these are due to lagophthalmos and dryness [3, 4].

In this case, the corneal abrasion was brought about by the excessive drying of the eye most likely due to antiphospholipid antibody syndrome. It is important to prevent this from happening. Personally I use saline and no ointment and/or lubricants. The latter can have side effects including blurry vision, erythema, and eye discomfort [5, 6]. Oil based eye ointment have also been known in one pediatric case to be explosive (Elliot Krane, personal communication 2008). I have had many patients complaining bitterly about blurry vision from oil based eye ointment postoperatively.

Recommendation

Patients with autoimmune dry eyes undergoing general anesthesia should have preventive measures to attempt to eliminate postoperative corneal abrasions.

References

1. Brock-Utne JG, Botz G, Jaffe RA. Perioperative corneal abrasions. Anesthesiology. 1992;77:221.
2. Kulkarni V, Lau G, Brock-Utne JG. Prevention of corneal abrasions in patients with autoimmune dry eyes. Anesth Analg. 2009;108:385–6.
3. Gild WM, Posner KL, Caplan RA, Cheney FW. Eye injuries associated with anesthesia. A closed claims analysis. Anesthesiology. 1992;72:204–8.

4. Batra YK, Bali IM. Corneal abrasions during general anesthesia. Anesth Analg. 1977;56: 363–5.
5. Siffring PA, Poulton TJ. Prevention of ophthalmic complications during general anesthesia. Anesthesiology. 1987;66:569–70.
6. White E, Crosse MM. The etiology and prevention of peri-operative corneal abrasions. Anaesthesia. 1998;53:157–61.

Chapter 24
Case 24: An Airway Surprise

You are called to the ICU for an airway problem. You arrive and find an 86 year old man who does not seem to want to stop coughing. The nurse said she had been encouraging him to take large breaths, when he suddenly started to cough. His oxygen saturation is 86% and he does not want the oxygen mask on his face. He is sitting up and looks like he is fighting for his life. He is holding onto his neck but cannot tell you what the problem is. He won't open his mouth.

He is in the ICU recovering from a removal of a subdural hematoma done 3 days ago. This he got after falling down some stairs at home.

The operation was done under local anesthesia which he tolerated well. You look at the anesthetic record which is noncontributory to the problem at hand.

You order a chest X-ray but really do not know what you are looking for. You are really at a loss as to what to do.

Question

What would you suggest?

J.G. Brock-Utne, *Case Studies of Near Misses in Clinical Anesthesia*,
DOI 10.1007/978-1-4419-1179-7_24, © Springer Science+Business Media, LLC 2011

Solutions

The chest X-ray shows a nasopharyngeal airway tube has slipped into the trachea and the tip is in the right main bronchus. You order an anesthetic machine and do an inhalational induction with sevoflurane in 100% oxygen. When the patient is asleep you remove the nasopharyngeal airway without difficulty using a MacIntosh blade and a Magill forceps. This is akin to a reported case report [1].

Previous studies have highlighted this problem. Several suggestions have been suggested as to how to secure the nasopharyngeal airway so that this does not occur [2–4]. Mobbs [2] has suggested a safety-pin be inserted at right angles through the proximal end of the airway thereby preventing dislodgement. However, the safety-pin hinders pharyngeal suction and the application of a T-piece for oxygen administration. Beattie [3] proposed to place an endotracheal tube connector/adaptor at the proximal end of the nasal airway. This prevents the migration of the nasopharyngeal airway, allows suction and the attachment of a T-piece. A modification of this technique has been described by Mahajan et al. [4].

Recommendation

The nasopharyngeal airway can migrate into the trachea causing coughing and severe distress to patients. This is worth remembering as this complication does occur.

References

1. Yokoyama T, Yamashita K, Manabe M. Airway obstruction caused by nasal airway. Anesth Analg. 2006;103:508–9.
2. Mobbs PA. Retained nasopharyngeal airway. Anaesthesia. 1989;44:447.
3. Beattie C. The modified nasal trumpet maneuver. Anesth Analg. 2002;94:467–9.
4. Mahajan R, Kumar S, Gupta R. Prevention of aspiration of nasopharyngeal airway. Anesth Analg. 2007;104:1313.

Chapter 25
Case 25: Difficulty with Breathing in the Postoperative Period

You are called to the recovery as a patient is complaining of difficulty in breathing. It is late in the day and you are on call. The anesthesiologist who had anesthetized the patient has gone home. In the recovery room you find a 28 year old woman who has undergone a robot-assisted salpingo-oophorectomy for an adnexal mass. Her past history is significant for hypertension, asthma (which is recorded in the preoperative note as not response to asthma drugs), and anxiety. She is 85 kg and 5 ft 9 in. The operative course and the first 10 min in the recovery room had been uneventful. The nurse tells you that she has suddenly now started complaining about difficulty in breathing. Her vital signs are HR 96 bpm, BP 160/96 and the oxygen saturation is 100%. A facemask with 10 L of oxygen is flowing through the mask. She states she cannot breathe and you can see that she is obviously very anxious. She tells you the tightness is not in her chest but in her throat. You note that her neck is a flexed position. You examine her and discover that she has an inspiratory stridor. She has no difficulty in speaking. There is no cough or sputum.

Not knowing what to do, you attempt racemic epinephrine with minimal improvement. Decadron, 10 mg and fursemide 20 mg IV does not have any effect. The chest X-ray you ordered in the recovery is normal. There is no hyperinflation or peribronchial thickening which you may see commonly with asthma.

Question

What can the diagnosis be and how will you suggest treating her symptoms?

J.G. Brock-Utne, *Case Studies of Near Misses in Clinical Anesthesia*,
DOI 10.1007/978-1-4419-1179-7_25,

Solutions

You do a fiberoptic laryngoscopy and note that the vocal cords are freely moving with paradoxical closing on inspiration (Seip LA, 2009, personal communication). A paradoxical vocal cord motion disorder (PVCM) is diagnosed [1].

PVCM is characterized by paradoxysmal periods in which the vocal cords adduction inspiration and/or expiration. This leads to a restriction of the airway causing dyspnea, wheezing, and/or stridor. This presentation can often be mistaken for asthma and the misdiagnosis for an individual patient may last for 15 years [2]. In many cases with acute presentation of PVCM there is unnecessary drug use, hospitalization, endotracheal intubations, and even tracheostomy [3].

The overall incidence of PVCM ranges from 2.8 to 12% [4, 5]. Psychogenic factors are considered major triggers for PVCM. The association between PVCM and asthma is unclear but there is a strong link between gastroesophageal reflux disease (GERD) and PVCM [6]. There have been reports that general anesthesia can cause PVCM [7]. A retrospective study has indicated that PVCM is generally a self-limiting disease, with few patients having long-term sequelae [7].

This case was successfully treated with a small dose of midazolam [8]. It is important however that one makes sure that the patient has not got CO_2 retention prior to giving a sedative drug.

The big differences between PVCM and asthma can be summarized as:

With PVCM it is more common in young females while asthma can occur at any age. The triggers for PVCM include stress, exercise, and general anesthesia while asthma has a multitude of triggers. The sensation of tightening in the throat is more common with PVCM than asthma as the latter has more signs of tightening of the chest. The inspiratory stridor is heard loudly over the larynx in PVCM, while this is very rare in asthma. Furthermore, PVCM patient rarely produce sputum, wake up at night with the symptoms, respond to asthma medication, and have an increase in residual volume. The chest X-ray is usually normal in PVCM while it is abnormal in asthma.

Recommendation

Remember PVCM may be a cause of respiratory distress in the recovery room, although not common.

References

1. Ibrahim WH, Gheriani HA, Almohamed AA, Raza T. Paradoxical vocal cord motion disorder; past, present and future. Postgrad Med J. 2007;83:164–72.
2. Morris MJ, Allan PF, Perkins PJ. Vocal cord dysfunction, aetiologies and treatment. Clin Pulm Med. 2006;13:73–86.

3. Maillard I, Schweizer V, Broccard A. Use of botulinium toxin type A to avoid tracheal intubation and/or tracheostom in severe paradoxical vocal cord movement. Chest. 2000;118:874–7.
4. Kenn K, WIller G, Bizer C. Prevalence of vocal cord dysfunction in patients with dyspnea. First prospective clinical study. Am J Respir Crit Care Med. 1997;155:A965.
5. Morris MJ, Deal LE, Bean DR. Vocal card dysfunction in patients with exertional dyspnea. Chest. 1999;116:1676–82.
6. Perkner JJ, Fennelly KP, Balkissoon R. Irritant associated vocal cord dysfunction. J Occup Environ Med. 1998;40:139–43.
7. Doshi DR, Weinberger MM. Long term outcome of vocal cord dysfunction. Ann Allergy Asthma Immunol. 2006;96:794–9.
8. Roberts KW, Crnkovic A, Steiniger JR. Post anesthesia paradoxical vocal cord motion successfully treated with midazolam. Anesthesiology. 1998;89:517–9.

Chapter 26
Case 26: Severe Systemic Local Anesthetic Toxicity

A 42 year old man (ASA 1) is scheduled for an elective elbow surgery. He is 72 kg and 6 ft). He consents to an interscalene block as he would prefer not to have a general anesthetic. In the preoperative holding area an IV is placed. Sedation, consisting of 2 mg midazolam and 50 mcg of fentanyl is given. The block is done in the following manner. The interscalene grove is identified at the level of C6 using a Stimuplex-DIG nerve stimulator (R. Braun, Inc., Bethlehem, PA 18018). The brachial plexus is identified by eliciting a biceps stimulation (0.1 ms duration, 2 Hz) 0.4 mA. A 40 mL solution consisting of (20 mL bupivacaine, 0.5% and 20 mL mepivacaine 1.5%) is injected slowly over a 2 min period. The patient is awake during the block. No blood or paresthesias is seen during the procedure.

Approximately 30–40 s after the needle is removed; patient becomes incoherent, stops breathing, and develops a tonic–clonic seizure.

Questions

1. What is your management of such a case?
2. When do you start lipid infusion immediately or when?

J.G. Brock-Utne, *Case Studies of Near Misses in Clinical Anesthesia*,
DOI 10.1007/978-1-4419-1179-7_26, © Springer Science+Business Media, LLC 2011

Solutions

To answer the second question first, lipid infusion should only be used after standard resuscitative measures have proven ineffective [1].

I have had six serious systemic reactions in 40 years. Five were caused by bupivicaine and one by lidocaine. Luckily all patients recovered without ill effects. They only remember a needle in some part of their body, before the "lights" went out.

The way I was taught and the way I handled all the earlier mentioned cases is summarized herein:

Since the patient is not breathing I give succinylcholine and rapidly place an endotracheal tube in the patient's trachea. Thereafter, I gave midazolam/thiopental to stop the seizing that is still going on in the brain. The object of securing the airway and ventilating the patient with 100% oxygen is to prevent respiratory acidosis. "Oxygen 8 L/min delivered by facemask attached to a self-inflating resuscitation bag" [2] will never reverse the severe respiratory acidosis which occurs within 30 s after tonic–clonic seizures [3–5]. In 1960 Moore and Bridenbaugh [6] reported 112 "Severe systemic reactions" (respiratory arrest, convulsions, cardiovascular collapse) in 36,113 patients from local anesthetics (amino-esters and amides) without mortality or morbidity. They [6] postulated that (a) with the onset of tonic–clonic seizures, severe respiratory acidosis occurred simultaneously i.e., within seconds and (b) effective oxygen therapy and maintenance of cardiac perfusion was the "antidote" to avoid severe, permanent complications from local anesthetics.

Moore and Bridenbaugh [6] have outlined how they avoid morbidity and mortality from seizures due to local anesthetics. I have taken the liberty to modify his proposal somewhat.

Before executing any regional block you must have:

1. Standard monitors placed on the patient. The same as you would do for any general anesthetic and/or monitored anesthesia care with sedation.
2. Immediately available drugs for resuscitation.
3. Immediately available endotracheal tubes and your favorite laryngoscope.
4. A working suction.

You notice that I have not included, as recommend by Weinberg [1], 20% lipid emulsion. He has recommended that the lipid be available in all operating room, block rooms, obstetric units, and other sites where local anesthetics are used including plastic surgery outpatients suites [1]. I totally disagree with him, as the infusion of lipid emulsion has only been shown to increase the survival rates in rats and dogs after an overdose of bupivacaine [7–9]. There are only two human case reports [2, 3] that claim successful resuscitation of local anesthetic-induced cardiovascular collapse. The one by Rosenblatt et al. [2] you should read. After that you should read all the letters to Anesthesiology that was published in March 2006 after Rosenblatt's case was published. If you do then you will understand that Rosenblatt's case report raises more questions than answers [6]. Recently, Hicks et al. [10] found that lipid emulsions combined with epinephrine and vasopressin does not improve survival in a swine model of bupivacaine-induced cardiac arrest.

Recommendation

When you are confronted with severe systemic local anesthetic toxicity, remember oxygen. The best way to safely give oxygen to an apneic patient is to secure the airway with an endotracheal tube.

I recommend you be undecided about the effectiveness of lipid emulsion, as a first line of defense, to successfully treat systemic bupivacaine toxicity.

References

1. Weinberg G. Lipid Infusion resuscitation for local anesthetic toxicity. Anesthesiology. 2006;105:7–8.
2. Rosenblatt MA, Abel M, Fisher GW, Itzkovich CJ, Eisenkraft CJ. Successful use of a 20% lipid emulsion to resuscitate a patient after a presumed bupivacaine related cardiac arrest. Anesthesiology. 2006;105:217–8.
3. Warren JA, Thoma RB, Georgescu A, Shah SJ. Intravenous lipid infusion in the successful resuscitation of local anesthetic-induced cardiovascular collapse after supraclavicular brachial plexus block. Anesth Analg. 2008;106:1578–80.
4. Moore DC, Crawford RD, Scurlock JE. Severe hypoxia and acidosis following local anesthetic-induced convulsions. Anesthesiology. 1980;53:259–60.
5. Moore DC, Thompson GE, Crawford RD. Long acting local anesthetic drugs and convulsions with hypoxia and acidosis. Anesthesiology. 1982;56:70–2.
6. Moore DC, Bridenbaugh LD. Oxygen: the antidote for systemic toxic reactions from local anesthetic drugs. JAMA. 1960;174:842–7.
7. Moore DC. Lipid rescue from bupivacaine cardiac arrest: a result of failure to ventilate and maintain cardiac perfusion? Anesthesiology. 2007;106:636.
8. Winberg G, VadeBoncouer T, Ramaraju GA, Garcia-Amaro MF, Cwik M. Pretreatment or resuscitation with a lipid infusion shifts the dose-response to bupivacaine-induced asystole in rats. Anesthesiology. 1998;88:1071–5.
9. Winberg G, Ripper R, Feinstien DL, Hoffman W. Lipid emulsion infusion rescues dogs from bupivacaine-0 induced cardiac toxicity. Reg Anesth Pain Med. 2003;29:198–200.
10. Hicks SD, Salcido DD, Logue ES, Suffoletto BP, Empey PE, Poloyac SM, et al. Lipid emulsions combined with epinephrine and vasopressin does not improve survival in a swine model of bupivacaine-induced cardiac arrest. Anesthesiology. 2009;111:138–46.

Chapter 27
Case 27: A Motorcycle Accident with Neck Injury

A 28 year old, 70 kg, 6 ft 1 in., male arrives in the emergency room (ER). He has fallen off his motorbike. You are called to come and assess him for general anesthesia as an abdominal tap has revealed free blood in the peritoneum.

You are told when you arrived in the ER, that the patient was unconscious at the scene for approximately 5–10 min. It is now 45 min since the accident and he is confused and mildly agitated. His past medical history is unknown. His vital signs are: HR 118 bpm and regular, BP 85/45 mmHg, respiration 28/min. temperature 36.5°C. His oxygen saturation is 95% on 10 L of oxygen delivered by face-mask. He has two 16 gauge catheters in each of his antecubital fossae.

On physical exam, you note several tattoos over his arms and torso. The patient is also on c-spine precautions, with a large cervical neck collar in place. An 8 cm forehead laceration is seen. His chest is clear to auscultation. There is no evidence of surgical emphysema on the anterior portion of his chest. His heart sounds are unremarkable, but distant. He moves all limbs. A chest X-ray shows no infiltrates, fractured ribs, subcutaneous emphysema, pneumo- or hemothorax.

You order two units of blood and accompany him to the CT scanner. The CT scan shows free blood in the peritoneal cavity and possible laceration of the liver. The patient is booked for an exploratory laparotomy for intra-abdominal hemorrhage secondary to a possible lacerated liver. Since the operating room is not ready the patient is taken back to the ER. While you go up the operating room to get ready, the ER physician places a subclavian venous catheter.

After 30 min the patient arrives in the operating accompanied by an ER nurse and an orderly.

J.G. Brock-Utne, *Case Studies of Near Misses in Clinical Anesthesia*,
DOI 10.1007/978-1-4419-1179-7_27, © Springer Science+Business Media, LLC 2011

Questions

There at least three important things for you to do prior to anesthetizing the patient in the operating room? What are they?

Solutions

Here are the things you must do prior to anesthetizing the patient:

1. Take off the cervical neck collar to examine his neck and chest for any evidence of: (a) subcutaneous emphysema. I know you did examine the chest in the ER but you could not have done the neck. In any case do it again. I can only tell you that things change. If surgical emphysema is present this is a serious warning sign of airway injuries, (b) any open wounds, (c) hematoma, (d) blunt injury to the neck, and (e) a concerning preoperative airway exam. If any abnormality is seen then you may be better off doing a fiberoptic intubation to secure the airway. If you do not remove a neck collar prior to anesthesia in a case like the one mentioned previously, then it could lead to disaster for the patient. I got involved, after induction of anesthesia, in a similar emergency case in which the neck collar was not removed prior to a rapid sequence induction. The discovery that it was neither impossible to ventilate nor intubate the trachea after the patient was asleep, led to an emergency tracheostomy. The case nearly ended in the demise of the patient.
2. Reexamine the chest by palpation, percussion, and auscultation one more time as the subclavian catheter insertion may have created a pneumothorax. If at all possible, I always insist the patient sit up. This so I can examine their back, not only to listen to the lungs but examine for tenderness (e.g., rib fractures) or observe discoloration and/or evidence of blunt trauma. The fact that in this case, the first chest X-ray did not reveal any lung pathology like a pneumothorax is no guarantee that it could not happen later or that the new subclavian vein insertion may have caused a pneumothorax. This scenario has happened to me and will happen to you if you are not vigilant.
3. Always check that all central lines are working prior to using them [1]. This is especially true, if you did not put the line in. Never trust anyone else's IV's. If you do, you will one day regret it.

Recommendation

Always take a patient's neck collar off to examine the airway properly.

Reference

1. Ottestad E, Schmiessing C, Brock-Utne JG, Kulkarni V, Parris D, Brodsky JB. Central venous access in obese patients. A potential complication. Anesth Analg. 2006;102:1293–4.

Chapter 28
Case 28: Thoracic Incisional Injury

A 28 year old, 80 kg 5 ft 10 in., male arrives in the emergency room by ambulance. He has been in a fight and has received a single 30 cm machete injury to his right chest. The incision extends from the right of the sternum at the level of T-6 towards the midaxillary line. His vital signs are stable – HR 100 bpm, BP 120/79, RR 30/min. You examine him carefully and discover no other injuries. He has no past medical history of note. You find him fully conscious but complaining of pain. His Hct is 28%. An IV is started and an intercostal chest drain inserted. The latter is seen to be working great, but a great deal of white-pink froth is also noted in the underwater seal bottle. The patient is taken to the operating room for exploration of the chest. The thoracic surgeon tells you there is no need for a double-lumen tube.

Questions

How would you anesthetize this patient? Would you consider a double-lumen tube, despite the surgeon's opinion? If so, why?

DOI 10.1007/978-1-4419-1179-7_28,

Solutions

You should consider a bronchopleural fistula due to the extent of the injury and the tremendous bobbling going on. The presence of the white-pink froth in the underwater drain is most like due to the hundreds of secondary or tertiary bronchioles cut during the attack with the machete, causing a clinical picture similar to that seen with a bronchopleural fistula.

In this case, which is similar to one previously described [1], a rapid-sequence technique was used with cricoid pressure. A left double-lumen was inserted into the trachea. Initially both lungs were ventilated, but the patient suddenly became cyanotic with an unrecordable oxygen saturation. The right lumen of the double-lumen tube ventilating the right lung was occluded by a clamp at the mouth end, leaving the only the left lung to be ventilated. The patient's color immediately improved and the oxygen saturation rose above 97%. A large single laceration of the lung, a 15 cm laceration of the diaphragm and 5 cm laceration of the liver were found. The diaphragm and the liver lacerations were repaired. The chest was closed. The right lung was seen to expand adequately, but again, when both lungs were ventilated the oxygen saturation fell precipitously. The patient's left lung was ventilated for the next 10 h and the vital signs remained stale. When he was able to ventilate spontaneously with both lungs via the double-lumen tube, it was removed. He continued to improve and was discharged from the hospital 4 days later.

Had a single lumen tube been used, a potential disaster could have occurred due to an inability to isolate the right lung quickly. The use of a double-lumen tube in a rapid-sequence technique in patients with airway classes 1 and 2 is not an added hazard to getting control of the airway. However, make sure you have at least two smaller double tubes in the room. The verification of the correct position of the tube can be done either with the Brodsky technique [2] or by using fiberoptic laryngoscopy [3].

Recommendation

When a bronchopleural fistula is suspected, a double-lumen tube is the right tube to use.

References

1. Naiker S, Brock-Utne JG, Aitchison J. Major thoracic incisional injury: ventilator management. Anesth Analg. 1989;68:702.
2. Brodsky JB (ed) (1990) Thoracic anesthesia. In: Problems in anesthesia. Lippincott, Philadelphia.
3. Berry F, editor. Anesthetic management of difficult and routine pediatric patients. New York: Churchill Livingstone; 1986. p. 167.

Chapter 29
Case 29: Bronchospasm – An Unusual Cause

A 4 year old child, 24 kg, is scheduled for a diagnostic upper endoscopy. Her major complaint is intermittent vomiting of unknown cause. Her medical history is significant for asthma. She takes nebulized albuterol, but only when needed. On physical exam you find nothing wrong and her lungs are clear to auscultation. On the day of surgery she is treated prophylactically with 2.5 mg nebulized albuterol and oral midazolam is given with good effect. At the patient's request an inhalation induction is performed using sevoflurane (up to 8% inhaled concentration) and 50% N_2O in oxygen. The patient falls asleep and an oral airway is inserted and positive-pressure ventilation is instituted by bag-mask ventilation with peak airway pressures of approximately 20 cm H_2O. You establish IV access and administer Lidocaine 36 mg (1.5 mg/kg) to prevent reflex bronchoconstriction caused by among other things endotracheal intubation [1]. Immediately after the lidocaine, the patient develops diffuse bilateral expiratory wheezes and a dramatic increase in peak inspiratory pressures. You discontinue N_2O and ventilate with sevoflurane in 100% oxygen. The oxygen saturation remains at 100% and the vital signs remain stable. No rashes or other signs of anaphylactic or anaphylactoid reactions are seen.

You are pleased that over a period of 5 min the wheezing resolves without further intervention and the peak pressure returns to 15 cm H_2O. An endotracheal tube was inserted uneventfully without the use of muscle relaxation. There was no further evidence of bronchospasm.

Question

What do you think the cause of the initial bronchospasm was?

J.G. Brock-Utne, *Case Studies of Near Misses in Clinical Anesthesia*,
DOI 10.1007/978-1-4419-1179-7_29,

Solutions

The most likely cause is the IV lidocaine [2]. Although IV lidocaine can, in humans, attenuate responses to inhalation challenges in awake subjects with airway hyperactivity [3], other studies have shown that the drug given IV constricts isolated airways [1, 4]. The reason for this is unknown [1].

The other cause of the sudden onset of airway problems could be related to a possible aspiration; however it is unlikely for wheezing etc. to resolve so quickly.

In this case [1], the rest of the anesthetic was uneventful with no further episodes of bronchospasm. The endoscopy exam was normal with no evidence of reflux or regurgitation.

Recommendation

IV lidocaine may cause airway narrowing in asthmatics.

References

1. Chang HY, Togias A, Brown RH. The effects o systemic lidocaine on airway tone and pulmonary function in asthmatic subjects. Anesth Analg. 2007;104:1109–15.
2. Burches BR, Warner DO. Bronchospasm after intravenous lidocaine. Anesth Analg. 2008;107:1260–2.
3. Groeben H, Schlicht M, Stieglitz S, Pavlakovic G, Peters J. Both local anesthetics and salbutamol pretreatment affects reflex bronchoconstriction in volunteers with asthma undergoing awake fiberoptic intubation. Anesthesiology. 2002;97:1445–50.
4. Downes H, Loehning RW. Local anesthestic contracture and relaxation of airway smooth muscle. Anesthesiology. 1977;47:430–6.

Chapter 30
Case 30: Post Bariatric Surgery – Any Concerns?

You are scheduled to anesthetize a 28 year old woman, 90 kg, 5 ft 7 in. tall, for abdominoplasty. Two years previously she underwent a laparoscopic gastric banding for morbidly obesity. Prior to that operation she was 188 kg. She now wishes to have excess abdominal skin removed. At this time she does not complain of gastroesophageal reflux, hypertension, and noninsulin dependent diabetes mellitus. Interestingly, she had these diagnoses prior to her gastric banding.

On the day of surgery she has neither eaten nor drunk anything for 12 h. You see her in the preoperative holding area. On examination you find nothing abnormal and classify her airway as class 2. An IV is easily placed and 2 mg midazolam IV has good effect. In the operating room you place standard noninvasive monitors.

Questions

Would you consider a rapid sequence in this patient? If, yes, why? If, no, why not?

J.G. Brock-Utne, *Case Studies of Near Misses in Clinical Anesthesia*,
DOI 10.1007/978-1-4419-1179-7_30, © Springer Science+Business Media, LLC 2011

Solution

You should always do a rapid sequence in a patient who has a past history of bariatric surgery. This is because there are detrimental changes in the anatomy and physiology of the gastrointestinal tract, including a decrease in esophageal-gastric peristalsis and impairment of lower esophageal sphincter relaxation [1, 2]. Furthermore, there is an increased risk of bronchial aspiration [3, 4] and increased possibility of aspiration pneumonia and long-term pulmonary complications [5] in these patients. Di Francesco et al. [6] showed that after a vertical banded gastroplasty, a decrease in basal lower esophageal sphincter tone and an increase in acid reflux also occurred.

It is interesting to note that in the study by Jean et al. [4], pulmonary complications were seen only in patients who had no premedication with H2-antagonists.

Recommendation

Patients who have had bariatric surgery are at risk for pulmonary aspiration and should be managed with a rapid sequence technique with cricoids pressure. Antacids, metoclopramide, and H2-antagonists should also be given.

References

1. Presutti RJ, Gorman RS, Swain JM. Primary care perspective on bariatric surgery. Mayo Clin Proc. 2004;79:1158–66.
2. Weiss HG, Nehoda HJ, Labeck B, Peer-Kuhberere MD, Klingler P, Gadenstatter M, et al. Treatment of morbid obesity with laprascopic adjustable gastric banding affects esophageal motility. Am J Surg. 2000;180:479–82.
3. Kocian R, Spahn DR. Bronchial aspiration in patients after weight loss due to gastric banding. Anesth Analg. 2005;100:1856–7.
4. Jean J, Compere V, Fourdrinier V, Marguerite C, Auquit-Auckbur I, Milliez PY, et al. The risk of pulmonary aspiration in patients after weight loss due to bariatric surgery. Anesth Analg. 2008;107:1257–9.
5. Alamoudi OS. Long-term pulmonary complications after laparascopic adjustable gastric banding. Obes Surg. 2006;16:1685–8.
6. Di Francesco V, Baggio E, Mastromauro M, Zoico E, Stefenelli N, Zamboni M, et al. Obesity and gastro-oesphageal acid reflex, physiopathological mechanism and role of gastric bariatric surgery. Obes Surg. 2004;14:1095–102.

Chapter 31
Case 31: Valuable Information from an Inplanted Pacemaker

Today you are anesthetizing a 68-year-old male, 84 kg and 5 ft 9 in., for a radical prostatectomy. To your dismay, you note that the surgeon doing the case is known for creating way above average blood loss. The patient has a history of coronary artery disease and hypertension. His HR is 70 bpm regular, BP 140/85, and oxygen saturation on room air is 97%. He claims his exercise tolerance is good, as he can walk two flights of stairs without stopping. On exam you discover a bulge under the patient's left collarbone. You ascertain that he has a pacemaker. There is no information about the pacemaker. The only thing the patient can tell you is that he has had it there for 3 years. He does not know why he got it. There is no information from the hospital records, as insertion was done at another hospital. As luck would have it, the Medtronic representative is in the preoperative holding area and you ask him to interrogate it. He tells you the battery is OK and that the pacemaker is set in a pacemaker dependent mode. Furthermore, he informs you that this is not an AICD (this is a device that delivers a direct current shock to the ventricle. The shock is in response to sensing ventricular fibrillation or ventricular tachycardia).

The Medtronic representative offers to reprogram the pacemaker to a NON-sensed mode like VOO (ventricular paced with no sensing and no inhibition) or DOO (Dual chambers (A&V) paced) mode for surgery at a rate of 70 bpm.

Questions

1. Will you agree to that?
2. Is there any other important information that can be extracted from the interrogation of the pacemaker?

DOI 10.1007/978-1-4419-1179-7_31,

Solutions

1. Since this may be a bloody mess, I would recommend you set the rate at 80 bpm in the DOO mode.
2. Most modern pacemakers have a feature that continuously monitors and records the underlying rhythm. This is called a Cardiac Compass Histogram. This histogram tells you type and frequency of arrhythmias that have occurred each day for the past 10 days.

In this case, we discovered to our dismay that this patient had been in and out of a new onset of atrial fibrillation for 4 days prior to the day of surgery. We canceled the surgery and sent him for a cardiology consult.

If the pacemaker is not pacer dependent, you can choose to either leave it alone or set it to asynchronous mode. For patients that just have the pacer for backup, it is better not to change anything. Just leave it. The patients should be able to increase their own rate in response to pain/hypovolemia/stress etc.

It is most important to remember to place the bovie pad far away from the device to minimize any interference. If, during the case, the heart rate slows down below the set rate of the pacemaker, the pacer will fire as it is supposed to but the bovie will interfere with the device's ability to recognize a need to fire. This can lead to cardiac pauses and dropped beats. If that happens, then the surgeon should only use short bursts of the cautery or change to a bipolar.

If you get in a jam with long cardiac pauses and excessive dropped beats, then you must put a magnet on the pacer. For most new devices (since 2006), a magnet puts the pacer in an asynchronous mode like DOO (Dual. No chamber or response to sensing) or VOO (Ventricle. No chamber (s) response(s) to sensing) at a rate of 80 bpm. You are now safe from bovie interference. Once you take off the magnet, it should go back to its prior setting DDD (Dual Chamber(s) sensed and usually response(s) to sensing).

Recommendation

Modern pacemakers have a cardiac compass histogram as a feature. This can tell you the underlying rhythm and any changes that have occurred in the recent past. This is important information for both you and the patient.

Chapter 32
Case 32: Allen's Test in an Anesthetized Patient – Is It Possible?

You are the anesthesiologist for a 62-year-old man, 60 kg and 5 ft 10 in., undergoing a Whipple procedure for pancreatic carcinoma. Two hours have elapsed and everything is going well and there is only minimal bleeding. Both arms are secured on arm boards at 80° to the operating table. With considerable dismay you notice that his right hand, in which you have placed a 20-gauge arterial catheter, is pale. This is a change from how it appeared prior to the radial artery cannulation. You discover that there is no capillary filling in his nail beds. Spasm/thrombosis is the most likely cause. There are two ways of dealing with this problem. (a) Leave the catheter in and warm up the hand with blankets at up to 45°C. If and when the hand shows capillary filling, you can take the catheter out. If the hand does not improve, it has been suggested that you can give lidocaine or vasodilator drugs through the catheter if you think this is a spasm. If it is a thrombus, you have a problem or (b) take the catheter out immediately. Unfortunately there are no prospective studies to show what the best options are.

In this case, you call a vascular surgeon. You follow his advice and take it out immediately. Ten minutes later, there is a lot of blood loss and therefore a need for an arterial line. You consider a left axillary or brachial artery line. But since you have never done one and have heard bad reports about them, you prefer to do a left radial artery cannulation. You want to do an Allen's test prior to inserting the radial artery cannula. But the problem is that the Allen's test requires the patient to be cooperative and he is not, as he is asleep and paralyzed.

Question

How would you attempt to determine the patency of the left ulnar artery intraoperatively prior to left radial artery cannulation?

J.G. Brock-Utne, *Case Studies of Near Misses in Clinical Anesthesia*,
DOI 10.1007/978-1-4419-1179-7_32, © Springer Science+Business Media, LLC 2011

Solution

Before answering the question, let us review the Allen's test [1]. The test evaluated flow from the radial and ulnar artery, occluding one vessel at a time. However, a modification of the Allen's test is now recommended [2]. In this test, the radial and ulnar arteries are compressed. The patient is asked to clench his fist until it blanches. The patient then relaxes the hand. Pressure on the ulnar artery is released. The skin should promptly become hyperemic, indicating that ulnar collateral flow is adequate. Unfortunately, the Allen's test is not predicative of ischemic damage after cannulation [3]. Others [4, 5] have suggested the use of strain gauge plethysmography to ensure adequacy of collateral flow to the hand or Doppler plethysmography [5].

The solution for the case above is to use the Brodsky's modification of the Allen's test [6]. A pulse oximeter is placed on the patient's thumb. You compress both radial and ulnar arteries resulting in the loss of pulse on the monitor. When, in normal patients, you release the pressure over the ulnar artery the pulse contour returns. If, on the other hand, this does not occur then this is a positive Brodsky sign. The beauty of this method is that it does not require patient cooperation, can be done without direct visualization of the hand (i.e., under the surgical drapes), and can be performed while the area is secured to an armboard. The results are objective and be more easily quantitated than those of the Allen's test.

In another case, I have seen a right index finger becoming pale following a right radial artery cannulation. The rest of the hand had a normal color. This was first noticed 20 min into the case. In that case, a separate oximeter was placed in the right index finger. It continued to read 100% for the rest of the 4 h operation. The right hand was warmed with an electric warming blanket. After 40 min, the finger returned to normal color. The arterial line was taken out in the recovery room and the right index finger was monitored continuously for the next 12 h. No desaturation or complications were seen. The patient was discharged home without any problem relating to the cannulation. The cause of the above problem was most probably spasm of the radial artery. The patient was told that in future, should he need an operation, he should inform the anesthesiologist of this event. This is the only time I have seen this in my 40 years of doing clinical anesthesia.

Recommendation

Remember the use of the Brodsky test to determine the patency of the ulnar artery intraoperatively prior to radial-artery cannulation.

References

1. Allen EV. Thromboangiitis obliterans: methods of diagnosis of chronic occlusive arterial lesions distal to the wrist with illustrated cases. Am J Med Sci. 1929;178:237–44.
2. Ghandi SK, Reynolds AC. A modification of Allen's test to detect aberrant ulnar collateral circulation. Anesthesiology. 1983;59:147–8.
3. Slogoff S, Keats AS, Arlund C. On the safety of radial artery cannulation. Anesthesiology. 1983;59:42–7.
4. Husum B, Palm T. Before cannulation fo the radial artery: collateral arterial supply evaluated by strain-gauge plethysmography. Acta Anaesthesiol Scand. 1980;24:412–4.
5. Morrayu JP, Brandford HG, Barnes LF, Oh SM. Doppler assisted radial artery cannulation in infants and children. Anesth Analg. 1984;63:346–8.
6. Brodsky JB. A simple method to determine patency of the ulnar artery intraoperatively prior to radial artery cannulation. Anesthesiology. 1975;42:626–7.

References

Chapter 33
Case 33: A Loss of the Only Oxygen Supply You Have During an Anesthetic

You are on an international medical trip. The operating room's only oxygen supply, an H-cylinder, is accidentally knocked over. This occurs in the middle of a general anesthetic in an otherwise healthy man. To your dismay you note that the regulator on the oxygen cylinder is so severely damaged, that oxygen is leaking out uncontrollably. A porter rushes in and takes the oxygen cylinder out of the room. He tells you that he will come shortly with a new one. Since the oxygen cylinder was the only fresh gas supply to the anesthesia machine (no piped oxygen, air or N_2O), the ventilation for the anesthetized and paralyzed patient ceased. The inhalational agent used was isoflurane. You look around and see no other oxygen source to continuously provide insufflations of oxygen. Furthermore, there is no facility to provide transtracheal jet ventilation, high frequency jet ventilation, transtracheal oxygen administration, intratracheal pulmonary ventilation, and tracheal gas insufflations.

You call for a self-inflating bag, an IV infusion pump to convert the anesthetic to an IV anesthetic, and a replacement for the damaged oxygen pressure regulator.

The hernia operation, in an ASA 1 male, is still 1 h away from being finished. Two minutes after the incident, the patient's vital signs remain stable with an oxygen saturation of 100%.

Question

While you wait, besides using your mouth to tube ventilation, what is the option or options you have at this time?

J.G. Brock-Utne, *Case Studies of Near Misses in Clinical Anesthesia*,
DOI 10.1007/978-1-4419-1179-7_33,

Solutions

This happened to a friend of mine, Lighthall [1]. The options he had were the following (a) hand ventilation through the functional carbon-dioxide-absorbing system. But the pop-off valve on the absorber must be closed quickly thereby minimizing the leak. This technique would dilute the alveolar anesthetic level, and the oxygen would disappear due to leaks in the circuit. Hence after a few minutes, it will be impossible to ventilate the patient. A better option (b) would be apneic oxygenation from a quiescent circuit [2]. In the latter, the exchange of gases between the blood and alveolar spaces is independent on the movement of gas to and from the lungs. Hence, oxygen for a time can be delivered to the circulation even if the patient is apneic. During apnea, negative pressure develops in the alveoli, because more oxygen is absorbed than CO_2 released. With the airway closed or obstructed, this will lead to a gradual collapse of the lungs. Since no CO_2 is removed from the alveoli, the partial pressure of CO_2 increases. Eventually, the CO_2 will displace oxygen and other gases from the airspaces and the patient will develop respiratory acidosis.

Lighthall [1] choose option (b) since this would most likely maintain alveolar anesthetic and oxygen levels longer than option (a). With (b) he could free his hands to prepare for an intravenous anesthetic. Therefore, further ventilation was suspended. Very clever was the fact that he disconnected the side-stream capnograph sampling line and capped it, so as not to waste oxygen from the circuit. The side-stream capnograph samples between 200 and 300 mL of fresh gas flow/min.

In the case described, the patient experienced 6–7 min of apnea and remained anesthetized with the oxygen saturation of 100%. He experienced no untoward effect and made an uneventful recovery.

Always insist on that a backup oxygen cylinder is present in the room. I remember working in remote hospital in Asia in about 1996. The hospital was very proud of the fact that they had piped oxygen. I wanted to see the oxygen source, but my hospital hosts refused to show me where it was located. They told me it would be of no interest to me. However one evening I sneaked out of my room in the hospital grounds and found it. The oxygen source was situated in a little shed (6×6 m). Inside, a man was sitting on a stool looking at the pressure gauge of a large oxygen cylinder. There was no oxygen production. Two large oxygen tanks were attached to the hospital pipeline. Only one tank was used at any one time. When the pressure gauge went to zero, the man quickly got up from his stool and activated the other cylinder, using a three-way-stop cock. The empty cylinder was quickly replaced and the man returned to his surveillance of the pressure gauge.

Recommendation

It is imperative to have an extra oxygen cylinder with its own functioning regular in the operating room. However, in these faraway places there may be no extra oxygen cylinders available as they are very expensive.

If you are caught in this situation, remember apneic oxygenation.

References

1. Lighthall GK. The value of simulation training during anesthesia residency. Anesthesiology. 2006;105:433.
2. Frumin MJ, Epstein RM, Cohen G. Apneic oxygenation in man. Anesthesiology. 1959;20:789–98.

Chapter 34
Case 34: An Aggressive Surgeon

This is your third day in a new hospital. You are assigned to do a general anesthetic for an 89-year-old woman (65 kg and 5 ft 8 in.) with an ingrown toenail on her left big toe. You meet the patient in the preoperative area. She arrives in a wheelchair, being pushed by her daughter. The daughter, who is a nurse, tells you that her mother is a "cardiac cripple," continuously in and out of congestive cardiac failure. The mother takes a large amount of cardiac medications including furosemide 80 mg twice a day. She has had several cardiac stents but unfortunately still gets angina at rest. Her exercise tolerance is poor as she becomes excessively breathless with angina even with dressing herself. When you meet her, she wants to talk only about her ingrown toenail. She has systemic hypertension and moderate pulmonary hypertension. She has stopped her Coumadin and her coagulation studies are normal. The note from the cardiologist tells you she is "stable." You are very concerned about a general anesthetic in this patient and suggest to the patient and daughter that the toe nail is best removed under a local block. The patient and daughter agree. You meet the surgeons, who you have never worked with before, and suggest a regional block of the toe. He does not like that idea and cannot understand what the problem is and says in an aggressive tone: "She has been cleared by cardiology for a general anesthetic. I don't have this problem with any of your other colleagues." Against your better judgment, you back down and agree to do a general anesthetic. The patient is taken to the operating room and standard monitors are placed. You give her no sedation. You record on your anesthesia record her vital signs as 86 bpm atrial fibrillation, BP 150/95, and oxygen saturation 92% on room air. You preoxygenate the patient and start a slow induction with etomidate. Your plan is to insert an LMA. The procedure should take no more than 5–10 min and you do not think a preoperative arterial line is indicated.

J.G. Brock-Utne, *Case Studies of Near Misses in Clinical Anesthesia*,
DOI 10.1007/978-1-4419-1179-7_34,

Question

Knowing that she is a high cardiac risk patient, what is it that you have forgotten to do in relation to the monitors?

Solution

You have forgotten to take a preoperative EKG strip from you anesthesia monitor. This case happened to me many years ago. Luckily I had been taught to do a preoperative EKG trace. That saved me and the patient. After approximately 4 mg of etomidate given over a 3–4-min period and with the patient still awake, her EKG showed sudden onset of ischemia. The surgeon was outside washing his hands at this time. When he came in, he discovered that the patient was not asleep and got very angry. I told him: "I am waking the patient up as she has had an ischemic event." He asked: "How do you know?" When I showed him the pre- and postinduction EKG, he was silenced. The case was done under local anesthesia. The patient had an uneventful anesthetic course. In the recovery room, a 12-lead EKG was unchanged when compared to the one after the insult. Blood was sent for troponium but came back negative. I informed the daughter of the event. On my insistence, the patient stayed 23 h postsurgery and was discharged home the next day.

Recommendations

1. Never get bullied into doing something that you know is wrong.
2. Always do a preoperative EKG strip in all patients who have a cardiac history. You will be pleased if you did.

Chapter 35
Case 35: A Pharyngeal Mass

Today you are scheduled to anesthetize a 3-year-old boy for pharyngoscopy and biopsy of a pharyngeal mass. The mother tells you the child has been healthy until this time. The present complaint is that he has become more breathless than normal, especially on exertion. On exam you note that his mouth opening is adequate, with good view of the uvula. His chest is clear and vital signs are normal except that the child is obviously somewhat distressed breathing even at rest. The A-P chest X-ray is normal and the lateral X-ray of the neck shows a large supraglottic soft-tissue mass. The mass projects from the posterior pharyngeal wall into the larynx which is narrowed by approximately 85%.

In the preoperative holding area, you establish an IV and take the child to the operating room. You call for the ENT surgeon and ask him to be ready to do an emergency tracheostomy. He agrees. You place the standard monitoring on the child and start an inhalational induction with sevoflurane in 100% oxygen. The inhalational anesthetic is well tolerated, but suddenly the airway muscle tone is lost and airway obstruction occurs. Repositioning of the jaw and head does not improve the obstruction, nor does the introduction of an oral airway. Your attempts at passing a small LMA fail. The patient's oxygen saturation falls and the sevoflurane is turned off. Luckily, the child awakens from the general anesthetic.

You now consider a tracheostomy under regional block with sedation but the surgeon is not happy with that idea. You are not happy either as you know that IV sedation, including ketamine, could cause irreversible airway obstruction. To add to your dilemma, the pediatric fiberoptic laryngoscope that is brought to you is found to be nonfunctioning and that is the only one in the hospital.

J.G. Brock-Utne, *Case Studies of Near Misses in Clinical Anesthesia*,
DOI 10.1007/978-1-4419-1179-7_35, © Springer Science+Business Media, LLC 2011

Question

What will you do now?

Solution

You attempt inhalational induction again with sevoflurane and 100% oxygen. Again, when the muscle tone is lost, airway obstruction occurs. This time however you grab the skin over the entire laryngeal cartilage and lift it and the larynx upward. The obstruction is immediately relieved. Spontaneous ventilation resumes and the anesthesia is deepened further. When anesthesia is considered to be adequate, laryngoscopy is performed and a supraglottic mass is seen overlying the glottis. A 3.5-mm i.d. uncuffed endotracheal tube (ETT) is passed into the trachea uneventfully. In this case, no oxygen desaturation occurred and no muscle relaxation was administered. The mass was biopsied and debulked. After return of consciousness, the ETT was removed with the patient in the right lateral position.

Recommendation

This simple technique should be tried when airway obstruction occurs during inhalational induction in patients with a supraglottic mass. It is imperative to be prepared for a respiratory disaster when dealing with cases like this. The surgeon must be in the room during anesthesia induction with his tracheostomy set at the ready.

Chapter 36
Case 36: Retained Laps

You have just completed an orthotopic liver transplant. It is late in the evening. Prior to closing, the instrument count revealed two missing laps. The OR staff conduct an extensive search and find one in the trash. The surgeon again examines the abdomen for the missing lap, but can't find it. Both an abdominal and chest X-ray is done in the OR. The radiologist calls into the room and states he can't identify any retained objects. The incision is closed and the patient is transported to the ICU. A routine chest X-ray taken, taken the next morning, shows clearly a retained lap in the upper abdomen.

Questions

How can this happen? Why was it not spotted last night in the operating room?

J.G. Brock-Utne, *Case Studies of Near Misses in Clinical Anesthesia*,
DOI 10.1007/978-1-4419-1179-7_36, © Springer Science+Business Media, LLC 2011

Solutions

In this case, the defibrillator pad obscured the lap pad's radio-opaque strip.
How do you prevent this from happening?

1. Always remove the defibrillator pad from the abdominal wall when looking for missing laps in the abdomen.
2. It is best to use radiolucent defibrillator pads (TZ Medical, Portland, OR 97224). These are marketed for intra-operative and ICU use.
3. Radiologist must communicate quality of film, bring hard copy to the OR for review by physicians, and if radiologists and/or the physicians are in doubt a repeat X-ray must be done.
4. Use only defibrillator pads in high-risk patients for arrhythmia.

When reviewing the literature [1], you find that the commonest cause of retaining foreign bodies is in elective, uncomplicated, and without change of scrub nurses shift. However, frequent explanations for retained laps are related to team fatigue, staff shifts with sloppy handovers, surgeon declines recount, false-negative X-ray, bloody procedures, and conversations in the OR.

I once worked with a surgeon who refused to have a chest X-ray to find a retained needle after a breast biopsy. She insisted it was on the floor. A magnet was brought in to find the needle but to no avail. I refused to wake the patient up until she had a chest X-ray. The needle was found in the chest wall in a 2 cm long incision. The surgeon said nothing.

Recommendation

Always remove the defibrillator pad from the abdominal wall when looking for missing laps.

Reference

1. Kaiser CW, Friedman S, Pfeifer Spurling K, Slowick T, Kaiser HA. The retained surgical sponge. Ann Surg. 1996;224:79–84.

Chapter 37
Case 37: A "Code Blue"

You are in the corridor outside many operating rooms when a nurse sticks her head out of one of the operating rooms and shouts: "We need you now." You run into the room. The room is very dark as a knee arthroscopy is taking place. The patient, you are told, is a 25-year-old healthy male football player, who has suddenly crashed. You can see that he is being ventilated with an endotracheal tube (ETT). All eyes are on the monitors. The vital signs are as follows; HR 140 bpm, BP and oxygen saturation are nonrecordable. There is no end-tidal CO_2, but a normal looking airway pressure wave form.

Question

What will you do?

J.G. Brock-Utne, *Case Studies of Near Misses in Clinical Anesthesia*,
DOI 10.1007/978-1-4419-1179-7_37, © Springer Science+Business Media, LLC 2011

Solutions

There are many things to do. As this happened to me I will tell you what I did.

1. I felt for the superficial temporal artery, just in front of the tragus of the ear. I could barely feel it. If you feel it, then the supine patient has at least 60 mmHg.
2. Next, I manually ventilated the lungs, listened with a stethoscope, and discovered bilateral air entry.
3. Disconnected the CO_2 sampling and blew into it, yielding a CO_2 trace.
4. Rechecked the superficial temporal artery for a pulse. Feeling none. I now reached for the epinephrine and gave nearly 1,000 μg of epinephrine.

The result was amazing. The oxygen saturation came back within seconds and so did the blood pressure albeit to 250/160 mmHg. You know this is short-lived but is there anything you can do to bring the BP down?

Turn on the vaporizer and the blood pressure will come down. I would not advice using a short-acting beta blocker.

The patient's vital signs stabilized and the surgery resumed. The cause of the very low BP was due to vancomycin 1 g having been given rapidly IV as a bolus dose causing "the red man syndrome."

The operation ends and the patient wakes up. What will you now do? He is an outpatient and wants to go home. Is that reasonable? No, this is what you must do:

1. Tell the patient what happened and advise him that he should stay a night.
2. Perform a 12-lead EKG in the recovery area, later that night and the next day morning.
3. Collect blood samples troponium for "rule out."

It is interesting to observe that these situations fortunately do not happen often in one's life as an anesthesiologist. Hence it is easy to say why I gave nearly 1,000 μg of epinephrine when 100 μg may have been sufficient. However, in my defense, you may only get one chance to give one epinephrine dose before you have a cardiac arrest. Hence make it work...

Recommendation

When faced with this sort of problem, remember ABC and the superficial temporal artery.

Chapter 38
Case 38: A Complication of Transesophageal Echocardiography

A 64-year-old physician (74 kg and 5 ft 11 in.) is scheduled to undergo an aortic valve replacement for aortic stenosis. He has a history of hypertension and smoking. Echocardiography has demonstrated an aortic valve area of 0.6 cm^2 and a mean pressure gradient of 66 mmHg across the stenotic aortic valve. Left ventricular hypertrophy is evident with normal systolic function and impaired diastolic function indicated by an abnormal relaxation pattern.

You see the patient in the preoperative area and place an IV and give him IV midazolam for sedation. In the operating room you place the routine monitors and induce anesthesia. Your resident places an endotracheal tube (ETT) in the trachea and confirms correct placement of the ETT. He also places an esophageal stethoscope/temperature probe in the esophagus. You, on the other hand, place an arterial line, while your resident now places a 7.5F pulmonary artery catheter (PAC) (Edwards Lifesciences, LLC, Irvine, CA). A normal pulmonary wedge pressure is obtained at a depth of 50 cm.

You tell the resident to place the transesophageal echocardiography (TEE). He is eager to do so; however, you now see something that he should do prior to inserting the TEE.

Question

What is it?

J.G. Brock-Utne, *Case Studies of Near Misses in Clinical Anesthesia*,
DOI 10.1007/978-1-4419-1179-7_38,

Solution

You must remember to remove the esophageal stethoscope/temperature probe in the esophagus prior to inserting the TEE. Failure to do so will cause serious complication [1]. In this case [1], a patient was admitted for anemia (HCT 19%) to a medical ward. Endoscopic evaluation for a presumed upper gastrointestinal bleed revealed small erosive lesions near the gastroesophageal junction (perhaps the cause of the low HCT) and a large tubular foreign body in the stomach. An attempt to remove it failed. It was later removed intact via a gastrotomy. The foreign body turned out to be an esophageal stethoscope. The likely explanation on how the esophageal stethoscope got there was that it was introduced during an aortic valve replacement 2 years before.

It is imperative to attach one's ear piece and/or the temperature probe once the esophageal stethoscope is in place. Had this been done, the above mishap as described in [1] would most likely have been prevented.

Recommendation

An esophageal stethoscope/temperature probe must always be attached to one's ear piece and/or temperature probe once the esophageal stethoscope is in place. In this way you should remember to remove it prior to the insertion of a TEE.

Reference

1. Brook M, Chard PS, Brock-Utne JG. Gastric foreign body: a potential risk when using transesphageal echo. Anesth Analg. 1997;84:1389.

Chapter 39
Case 39: LMA in Elective Orthopedic Surgery

A 25-year-old man is scheduled for an intramedullary nailing for a femoral fracture. He is otherwise healthy. One week before, he had a motor vehicle accident. Initially, he was treated conservatively, in the hospital, by sustained traction with the left leg in a Thomas's splint. But since a satisfactory reduction could not be secured by this method, surgery was recommended and accepted.

You met the above patient, as the first case of the day, in the preoperative area. He is 80 kg and 6 ft. He denies having had any food or liquid since midnight. The family is there and concurs as they are now going to have a big breakfast. You place one 18 G IV in his hand and reckon that you will not need any more IV access. The case is booked for 1 h. In the operating room you place standard monitors and induce anesthesia uneventfully. When the patient is asleep without using manual ventilation with vapor, an LMA is inserted easily with a leak at 20 cm H_2O. The surgeon wants the operating table up as high as it can go. This is done so he can stand and work on the femur. Sterile surgical drapes are placed over the patient, including his head. The surgery starts and everything is going well with the patient breathing spontaneously on nitrous oxide 70% in oxygen and sevoflurane. You titrate meperidine to a respiratory rate of 8–12 bpm. You sit down on your stool and start charting. The patient cannot be seen as he is lying on the operating table at least 3 ft above you. The vital signs are stable until you notice that the oxygen saturation falls from 98 to 92% over a period of 5 min. All the other vital signs are normal except that the peak airway pressures are increased from 18 to 28 cm H_2O. You now notice that the respiratory rate is also increasing and the tidal volumes are decreasing. Standing up, you close the APL valve on the anesthesia machine. You attempt to ventilate manually through the LMA. However, there is a definite increase in airway resistance, since you did the leak test about 35 min ago. You now take the surgical drapes off the head of the patient. The patient's chest is obviously heaving and you discover to your horror that there are undigested burritos etc. in the LMA. The oxygen saturation is now 89% and falling.

J.G. Brock-Utne, *Case Studies of Near Misses in Clinical Anesthesia*,
DOI 10.1007/978-1-4419-1179-7_39, © Springer Science+Business Media, LLC 2011

Question

What will you do now?

Solution

You call for help and inform the surgeon that you must put the operating table down and in steep Trendelenburg. Succinylcholine 1 mg/kg is given IV and an assistant applies cricoid pressure. When relaxation occurs, you disconnect the anesthesia breathing system at the elbow just above the LMA. Suction is applied to the proximal orifice of the LMA and it is removed quickly. You insert your laryngoscope and suction out his pharynx. Then you insert an endotracheal tube (ETT) into the patient's trachea and blow up the cuff. Before ventilation is commenced, you suck out as much as you can from the trachea. This case happened to a resident (Einar Ottestad) and I. The surgery was concluded uneventfully. In the recovery room, a chest X-ray was normal. He was admitted to a monitored bed. The next day he was discharged to an orthopedic ward. His vital signs remained stable with no evidence of aspiration pneumonia. A few days later, he is discharged home.

After the anesthetic, the parents and girlfriend were told about the complication. In this case, the patient later admitted that he had a full breakfast. His girlfriend had brought it in to hospital without anyone knowing it. The parents were horrified, while the girlfriend did not really understand the fuss.

It is interesting to speculate what would have happened if, after the IV induction, the patient would have been ventilated for a few minutes with oxygen and sevoflurane. The introduction of air into the stomach, by mask ventilation, thereby increasing intragastric, could have led to earlier regurgitation of the burritos etc. prior to the insertion of the LMA.

It is important to remember that regurgitation of stomach contents is more common than vomiting and just as hazardous.

Recommendation

Be prepared for aspiration with an LMA. If it does occur, rapid intervention will save the day. In this case, there were no signs that could have predicted this aspiration. However, it is a good idea to be suspicious and prepared for anything. One of my teachers once said to me: "Remember John, many, if not all patients lie."

Chapter 40
Case 40: What Would You Do?

You are a clinical professor of anesthesia, aged 54, working in a large university hospital. Since 7 a.m. you have been in the operating room supervising anesthetic cases. The time is now 5:30 a.m. the next day. You find yourself in the ICU to pick up a 4-year-old child who has been in a motor vehicle accident. He was an unrestrained passenger in the back seat. He is scheduled to have his facial laceration fixed by a plastic surgeon. The surgeon is anxious to get this case done prior to the start of his elective plastic list at 7:30 a.m. today. The case is booked for 1 h.

You examine the child and find that he has no other injuries. The mother and father are at the bedside. The mother tells you that the child has been healthy all his life. He has had no previous surgeries. The family histories of previous anesthetics are noncontributory. You ask the parents if they have any questions. The mother looks at you and asks: "How many hours have you been working continuously today?" You tell her that you have been giving anesthesia for 22.5 h. She looks at you and says: "You look exhausted." You assure her that you are OK and that the child will be safe in your care. However, you feel that you have not convinced her or her husband, nor do you like this extra pressure.

Questions

What are your options? You can refuse to do the case? Do the case? Delay the case? Get someone else to do the case later that day? What would you do?

J.G. Brock-Utne, *Case Studies of Near Misses in Clinical Anesthesia*,
DOI 10.1007/978-1-4419-1179-7_40,

Solution

This happened to me. I phoned the surgeon and told him about my interaction with the parents. Initially, he was not sympathetic and asked for another anesthesiologist. I told him that I was the only one. I then told him: "We all, including the patient and the family, would be better served with a new anesthesia team doing the case any time during your elective schedule today." He reluctantly agreed and I was able to tell the parents that child would be done later today with a new fresh anesthesia team. They were visually delighted. I informed the ICU nurse and told them not to feed the child.

Recommendation

Be acutely aware of the concern/need of patients/relatives prior to anesthesia. Always do the right thing whenever possible. The fact that this was an elective case and not an emergency made the delay of the case no problem, except some inconvenience for the surgeon.

Chapter 41
Case 41: Preeclampsia

You are in the labor and delivery suite as the attending anesthesiologist. It is late at night. You are asked to speak to a patient, with borderline preeclampsia, for a possible epidural. On entering the room, you find a 28-year-old primigravida who is otherwise healthy. She is alone except for a midwife. The midwife has recently come on duty and tells you that the previous midwife had just started an infusion of magnesium sulfate. You note that there are two Lactate Ringer IV bags (1,000 mL) hanging and one has "Magnesium" written on it. The patient is grateful and excited about the prospect of an epidural and gladly signs the consent form. You note that the patient has a good IV running with a hardly used unlabeled 1,000 mL Lactate Ringer. You ask the midwife to give the patient a preload with 500 mL of Lactated Ringer while you get ready to do the epidural. When ready you place the patient in left lateral position. You quickly perform the epidural and tread the epidural catheter. A test dose is given and you are happy to note no increase in the heart rate. You ask the patient if she can move her legs but she is very quiet and looks very comfortable. The oxygen saturation monitor has fallen off her finger and you ask the midwife to replace it. To your dismay, the oxygen saturation is 85% and falling. You look at the patient and recognize that she is cyanotic and would seem not to be breathing. You have injected nothing, either through the IV or the epidural catheter, except the test dose. The IV is running wide open and nearly 800 mL of the Lactated Ringer has now gone in. The midwife says she has not injected anything into the IV. The oxygen saturation is now 80%. You now notice that the fetal monitoring had been discontinued during the epidural.

Questions

What are you going to do? Why has the patient stopped breathing?

J.G. Brock-Utne, *Case Studies of Near Misses in Clinical Anesthesia*,
DOI 10.1007/978-1-4419-1179-7_41, © Springer Science+Business Media, LLC 2011

Solutions

You ask the midwife to perform cricoid pressure. From the emergency cart you grab an endotracheal tube (ETT) and a laryngoscope. An emergency cart should always be with the epidural cart. You don't move the patient from her lateral position but quickly secure the airway in this patient with an ETT. It is relatively easy to intubate the trachea with a patient in the left lateral position, as compared to the right lateral. This is because the tongue is falling way from the right side of the pharynx. In these cases you should not mask ventilate with 100% oxygen. It can prove dangerous, as these patients can aspirate. Leaving the patient in the left lateral position maintains maximum left uterine displacement. As soon as you have brought the oxygen saturation to 100% with an AMBU bag, you ask to midwife to connect the fetal monitor. You are happy to note that the baby is fine.

So how could this have happened? You disconnect the nearly empty Lactated Ringer fluid bag and the other one with the magnesium written on it and send them both to the laboratory for analyses of magnesium. The fluid bag is replaced with a new Lactated Ringer. Many hours later you are told that you were right in your suspicion. There was excess magnesium in the Lactated Ringer that you gave as a preload. The magnesium sulfate had been placed in one IV fluid bag and not labeled "Magnesium."

In high doses, magnesium will act as nondepolarizing muscle relaxant. This was what occurred in this case. The unlabeled IV fluid bag had magnesium sulfate drip in a concentration of 40 mg/mL. The other labeled bag had no magnesium in it. The preloading of the patient with the IV bag with magnesium raised the magnesium concentration from therapeutic levels of approximately 4–8 mEq/L to paralyzing levels of 10–15 mEq/L.

This case happened to me. The patient made an uneventful recovery and had no recall of what happened. A healthy baby boy was later delivered.

Recommendations

1. Magnesium sulfate has been shown to be effective in preventing grand mal seizures of eclampsia. But it is important to be aware of the dangers associated with its use. When using the drug, the IV bag with the magnesium must be clearly labeled. To do otherwise is to look for trouble.
2. You must always have standard resuscitative measures readily available when working in a labor and delivery ward. Things can happen very quickly, but if you are prepared for respiratory/cardiac arrests, then it is so much easier. You don't want to be caught like a carpenter without his tools. Always be prepared.

Chapter 42
Case 42: A Failed "Test Dose"

A 58-year-old morbidly obese patient is scheduled for an open gastric bypass. His past history is significant for hypertension and insulin-dependent diabetes with retinopathy. His medications include insulin, antihypertensive medication, and 0.5% timolol eye drops. You review the laboratory results and find them normal except that the blood glucose is elevated to 145 mg/dL. His EKG is normal. A dobutamine stress echocardiogram shows normal function of the left ventricle. His vital signs are normal and you place an IV in the preoperative area. The patient is taken to the OR and in a sitting position a single orifice epidural catheter is placed at a low thoracic level without difficulty. The catheter is estimated to be 5 cm in the epidural space. Initial aspiration reveals no cerebrospinal fluid (CFS) or blood. With the patient lying down, you administer a test dose (5 mL) containing 75 mg lidocaine with epinephrine 25 μg. The test dose is negative as there are no changes in the heart rate (HR) or ECG tracing. However, his BP increases from 165/78 to 185/88 mmHg. You aspirate the epidural catheter again and get back a tiny amount of blood-tinged fluid (<0.1 mL). You would like to use the epidural during the surgery but you are not sure if the catheter is intravascular. A repeat test dose gives the same result as above, no change in the ECG but a similar increase in BP. The surgeon is getting agitated and you decide to induce general anesthesia and not to use the epidural during surgery.

Questions

1. If the epidural catheter is intravascular why are there no ECG changes?
2. What other test can you do intraoperatively to establish if the catheter is indeed intravascular?
3. The patient arrives in the recovery room. Besides placing a new epidural what else can you suggest to do with the original epidural catheter?

J.G. Brock-Utne, *Case Studies of Near Misses in Clinical Anesthesia*,
DOI 10.1007/978-1-4419-1179-7_42,

Solutions

1. The systemic bioavailability of 0.5% timolol eye drops is nearly 80% [1]. Timolol eye drops have been shown to significantly reduce the HR increase caused by isoproterenol [2]. Hence patients who use ophthalmic timolol the night before surgery will not have an increase in HR following IV epinephrine [3].
2. By administering IV epinephrine intraoperatively, you can ascertain if you get the same HR rate response as you would with an intravascular epidural catheter. In the case by Bai-Han and Bradshaw [3], there was no increase in HR due to the timolol. In their case report [3], they showed that intravascular administered epinephrine failed to elicit tachycardia in a patient using timolol eye drops.
3. In the recovery room, you should pull back the epidural catheter by about 2 cm and repeat the test dose. In the case reported by Bai-Han and Bradshaw [3], the recovery room test dose led to no change in HR and BP. This suggested that the original epidural placement was indeed intravascular. The authors [3] then injected bupivacaine through the epidural catheter and produced a bilateral sensory loss in corresponding dermatomes.

Recommendation

Do remember that beta-receptor antagonist eye drops may block the beta-agonist effect of epinephrine given as an epidural test dose.

References

1. Berlin I, Marcel P, Ussan B. A single dose of three different ophthalmic beta-blockers antagonize the chronotropic effect of isoproternol in healthy volunteers. Clin Pharmacol Ther. 1987;41:622–6.
2. Stewart WC, Stewart JA, Crockett S. Comparison of the cardiovascular effects of unoprostone 0.15%, timolol 0.5% NS placebo in healthy adults under exercise using a treadmill test. Acta Ophthalmol Scand. 2002;80:272–6.
3. Bai-Han L, Bradshaw P. Intravascular administered epinephrine, injected inadvertently as part of an epidural test dose, failed to elicit tachycardia in a patient using timolol eye drops. Anesth Analg. 2007;104:1308–9.

Chapter 43
Case 43: A Simple Cystoscopy with Biopsy

A 73-year-old female (65 kg and 5 ft 10 in.) is scheduled for a cystoscopy. Her past history is unremarkable except for chronic interstitial cystitis. The patient has had numerous anesthetics for the above complaint. The family history is negative for anesthesia-related complications. The patient is taking no medication at present and is classified as an ASA 1. She requests an epidural anesthetic, and as there are no contraindications, an epidural is placed in L3–L4 interspace. Lidocaine 2% (15 mL) produces a good block, and the operation proceeds uneventfully. She does not want any sedation, so you don't give her any. As per the surgeon, she does not receive any antibiotic. Thirty-five minutes from the start of the surgery and while you are talking to her about her grandchildren, she suddenly says: "Doctor, I don't feel too good." You note that the ECG shows a sudden onset of ventricular tachycardia and the Dynamap alarms, indicating no blood pressure reading. The oxygen saturation has dropped from 100 to 76% over 1–2-min period. She has been receiving 2 L oxygen via a nasal cannula. You have given her no medication except for the lidocaine in the epidural space. The patient is now unconscious and, although you do not know what happened, you quickly place a face mask with 100% oxygen and assist her respiration. The superficial temporal artery cannot be palpated and the carotid pulse is very weak (see more discussion on this in Chap. 37). With the help of mask ventilation, the oxygen saturation has increased to 86% but she still has a weak carotid pulse and the Dynamap still alarms indicating no blood pressure can be measured. You call for a defibrillator and proceed to deliver a shock at 100 J. There is a rapid return to sinus tachycardia and the BP returns to normal as does the oxygen saturation. The patient complains of pain in the chest and looks at you upset and says: "What happened doctor? I have such a pain in my chest. What did you do to me and I thought you were a nice doctor." You say you are sorry and are at a loss to explain the cause of this event. You dismiss a toxic dose of systemic lidocaine as very unlikely.

J.G. Brock-Utne, *Case Studies of Near Misses in Clinical Anesthesia*,
DOI 10.1007/978-1-4419-1179-7_43,

Question

What is the possible cause of this sudden turn of events in an otherwise normal anesthetic?

Solution

In this case which happened to me, the surgeon eventually admitted that he injected epinephrine (1,000 μg) into the bladder wall. This was done to establish hemostasis.

When unexplained vital signs change from a baseline, it is important to make certain that you have not done anything that could be the cause of the problem. Having exhausted all your causes, it is time to ask the surgeon.

The surgeon and anesthesiologist should always keep each other informed during the intraoperative period, if they are doing anything that can alter the vital signs. If the surgeon in this case had told the anesthesiologist about the excess bleeding in the bladder and then inquired about the appropriate dose of epinephrine, this problem could have been avoided.

Recommendation

Surgeons should always inform the anesthesiologist about the drug concentration and the amount he/she is giving intraoperatively. If you see a surgeon inject anything into an anesthetized patient, under your care, it is your duty to enquire what it is and how much.

Chapter 44
Case 44: An Orthopedic Trauma

You are called to the emergency room where a 45-year-old man is admitted. He is morbidly obese and has sustained massive fractures to his pelvis and long bones after falling off his motor bike at great speed. Luckily, he was wearing his helmet while his female friend did not. She was dead on arrival to the hospital. You examine him and concur that he has no chest or head injury. He has very difficult IV access and the emergency doctor has placed an Arrow-Flex sheath (9Fr) (international, Reading, PA 19605) in his femoral vein. Colloid and crystalline solutions have been given and his vital signs are HR 100, BP 100/60. The orthopedic surgeon wants to take him to the operating room stat. You decide to secure the airway in the emergency room. You "ramp him up" for optimum tracheal intubating conditions [1] and secure the airway with etomidate and succinylcholine. The patient is transported to the operating room where a long and complicated orthopedic procedure commences. However, before the surgery starts, the groin sheath is removed since the surgeon does not want any interference with blood flow to the legs. You insert another Arrow Sheath in his right internal jugular. Another IV (16G) is inserted into a vein in his left forearm. The operation turns bloody. After 6 h he has been transfused 44 units of red blood cells with fresh frozen plasma and platelets. He is now on a neosynephrine drip to keep his blood pressure adequate. The operation finishes and he is to be transported to the ICU with full ventilator support. On moving this massive man from the OR table to the ICU bed, all IVs are accidently pulled out except the arterial line. You have been holding onto the endotracheal tube and head and were assured by the "moving team" that all lines were clear and no problem.

J.G. Brock-Utne, *Case Studies of Near Misses in Clinical Anesthesia*,
DOI 10.1007/978-1-4419-1179-7_44, © Springer Science+Business Media, LLC 2011

Question

The blood pressure falls precipitously. What are the options you do to quickly get the blood pressure back to more normal levels?

Solutions

You have actually three options:

1. Intra-arterial injection of epinephrine, but not neosynephrine. Epinephrine was used in this case. Bolus injections of epinephrine 100 μg kept the blood pressure within normal limits until new IVs were inserted. The patient was taken to the ICU. After 4 days, he was transferred to a regular ward and eventually home. He had no apparent complication from our fiasco.
2. Endotracheal injection of epinephrine. However, a study has shown that current recommended doses of epinephrine, administrated endotracheally (2 times the IV dose), are rarely effective in the setting of cardiac arrest and CPR [2]. I remember having an adult elderly patient who after induction of anesthesia developed severe bronchospasm. At the same time, I lost the only IV I had in the patient. The bronchospasm was only broken after 6,000–8,000 μg of epinephrine was given via the endotracheal tube. However, after we broke the bronchospasm we had a heart rate of over 130 for a long time.
3. Intraosseous infusion. Intraosseous seems to be faster and more reliable than the endotracheal tube [3–5]. Intraosseous infusion is used widely in children with good results [4, 5].

Recommendation

An arterial line can be used to give epinephrine if needed to maintain the vital signs.

References

1. Collins JS, Lemmens HJM, Brodsky JB, Lemmens HJM, Brock-Utne JG, Levitan RM. Laryngoscopy and morbid obesity a comparison of the "sniff" and the "ramped" positions. Obes Surg. 2004;14:1171–5.
2. Niemann JT, Stratton SJ. Endotracheal versus intravenous epinephrine and atropine in out-of-hospital "primary" and postcountershock asystole. Crit Care Med. 2000;28:1815–9.
3. LaRocco BG, Wang HE. Intraosseous infusion. Prehosp Emerg Care. 2003;7:280–5.
4. Isbye DL, Nielsen SL. Intraosseous access in adults – an alternative if conventional vascular access is difficult. Ugeskr Laeger. 2006;168:2793–7.
5. Dubick MA, Holcomb JB. A review of intraosseous vascular access: current status and military application. Mil Med. 2000;165:552–9.

Chapter 45
Case 45: Blood in the Endotracheal Tube

Today you are doing a repair of an aortic stenosis in a 58-year-old man (84 kg and 5 ft 11 in.) under cardiopulmonary bypass. You are going off bypass when you notice bright red blood filling your endotracheal tube (ETT). You suction the ETT, but the fresh blood keeps coming. In a period of 2–3 min, 100 mL of blood is collected in your suction canister. The patient's oxygen saturation falls and both the end-tidal CO_2 and the airway pressure rise. It is now impossible to ventilate the patient.

You order the patient back on bypass. This occurs uneventfully. Since the ETT is so bloody, you replace it. With the patient's blood pressure at a lower level, the bleeding stops. The total amount of blood from the ETT is now 600 mL. You insert a fiberoptic scope to attempt to ascertain the origin of the bleeding, but see no suspicious area.

Question

What will you do to try and establish the source of the bleeding into the bronchial tree and how will you stop it?

J.G. Brock-Utne, *Case Studies of Near Misses in Clinical Anesthesia*,
DOI 10.1007/978-1-4419-1179-7_45, © Springer Science+Business Media, LLC 2011

Solution

Ask the bypass technician to slowly go off bypass, while you examine the bronchial tree for the source of the bleeding. In this case, the bleeding was seen in the right bronchus below the carina and just below the takeoff of the right middle lobe. The bypass was ordered on and off over a period of 10–15 min. This was done to identify and to correctly place a bronchial blocker to prevent any further bleeding. The patient was taken to the ICU in a stable condition. Three days later, his right lower lobe was removed uneventfully at surgery. The patient was discharged home 10 days later.

Airway hemorrhage is classified as small (<15 mL blood), moderate (>15–30 mL), or large (continued blood loss) like in this case. In this case, the problem was caused by the surgeon who nicked the bronchial artery. The systemic bronchial artery causes more massive airway bleeding than the low-pressure pulmonary artery system. Carcinoma, lung disease, bronchiectasis, trauma, and postsurgical bleeding are the most common causes.

If this had happened in a patient not on cardiopulmonary bypass, the management would be different. With a double lumen, you can clamp ETT lumen to the bleeding lung. If on the other hand you had a single lumen tube then you could, if you were sure this was a right bronchial tear, push it or a smaller ETT blindly down the right main bronchus. By blowing up the ETT cuff, a tamponade effect should hopefully arrest the bleeding. With the bleeding under control, one should be able to ventilate the right lung.

The most common cause of massive pulmonary hemorrhage is pulmonary artery rupture from pulmonary artery catheterization. This complication is more likely to occur in patients who are older or have clotting defects or pulmonary hypertension. It also occurs when the catheter is placed distally and the balloon hyperinflated. If the pulmonary hemorrhage is caused by the pulmonary artery catheter, then it should be withdrawn centrally and not inflated. IPPV with or without PEEP may tamponade the bleeding. Reversal of anticoagulants and/or treatment of an underlying clotting problem if present should be instituted [1].

When airway hemorrhage occurs, it is imperative to isolate the normal lung quickly. This may be done with a double lumen tube or a single lumen as described above. Bronchoscopy (both rigid and fiber-optic) should be used to clear the airway, localize the bleeding and controll it. Passing a rigid bronchoscope is easy even if you have not done one previously. Just use your laryngoscope to place the bronchoscope. To the ENT surgeon, who most likely is not there, this is not the "correct" way to do it. But who cares. Once the normal lung has been protected from aspiration and the patient is deemed operable, a definite surgical treatment can commence. In those patients who continue to bleed and can't have surgery, selective bronchial arteriography and therapeutic embolization of the bronchial artery may be the solution. The latter must again be done when there is active bleeding so the radiologist can see the source of the bleeding. Embolization of the bronchial artery should not be taken lightly as the first branch of the bronchial artery goes to the spinal cord. If the bronchial artery flow gets compromised, then the spinal cord may be damaged.

Recommendation

Bleeding in the airway can be a disaster. It is important to keep calm, keep oxygenating the patient, and protect as much lung tissue as you can.

Reference

1. Ghosh S, Latimer RD. Thoracic anaestesia. Principles and practice. Oxford: Butterworth-Heinemann; 1999. p. 241–44.

Chapter 46
Case 46: A Longstanding Tracheostomy

A 3-year-old child has been in the ICU for 1 month. She has a tracheostomy and is breathing spontaneously. The tracheostomy is kept in place by a tie around her neck. She was involved in a major trauma and sustained a head injury, hemothorax, and lacerated liver. She is now scheduled for a laparotomy for the exclusion of possible sepsis in the abdomen.

The child is breathing with a tracheostomy mask (Hudson RCI, Teleflex, NC 27709). This mask is attached to a nebulizer with air entrainment and immersion heater adaptor (Cardinal Health, McGraw Park, IL 60085). Her chest is clear. The mother tells you that the patient has a "shelf" in her trachea. You ask her what that means. She tells you that she was told this by the ENT doctor after they had examined the child's trachea with a fiberscope. But the surgeon had told her: "This is nothing to worry about." You look in the notes but cannot find a note from the ENT doctors. You reexamine the child and find nothing wrong with either the tracheostomy or the chest. With the help of an orderly, you transport the patient to the operating room. Routine monitors are placed and your breathing circuit is attached to the tracheostomy. Good tidal volumes are recorded. An uneventful IV induction with vecuronium follows. As the patient is going to sleep, the surgeon sutures the tracheostomy to the skin. After 1–2 min you place the child on the ventilator but notice to your dismay that the peak airway pressures are over 55 cm H_2O. You attempt to manually ventilate the patient but find it difficult to move any air. You listen to the lungs. Prolonged inspiratory and expiratory wheezes are heard. You pass a suction catheter, with some difficulty, through the tracheostomy. There is nothing to suction. You try bronchodilators, but to no avail. The oxygen saturation has been falling slowly and is now 79%.

J.G. Brock-Utne, *Case Studies of Near Misses in Clinical Anesthesia*,
DOI 10.1007/978-1-4419-1179-7_46, © Springer Science+Business Media, LLC 2011

Question

What is your next step?

Solution

You quickly undo the sutures to the tracheostomy tube. You had noticed that the tracheostomy tube was pulled upward with the suturing. When the tracheostomy tube was placed more distal into the trachea, there was an immediate improvement in the airway pressure. The chest was now clear. You tell the surgeon about the "shelf." Using a fiberoptic scope, you ascertain that there was a large granulation tissue that obstructed 80% of the tracheal lumen. This explained the problem created when the tracheostomy tube was pulled more proximal in the trachea, putting the shelf into a position to occlude the tracheostomy tube.

Recommendation

A mother's concern should always be taken seriously. It is imperative to find out all you can about any potential problems, especially if it relates to the airway.

Chapter 47
Case 47: An Airway Problem During Monitored Anesthesia Care

A 48-year-old female (84 kg, 5 ft 8 in.) is scheduled for a rectal exam under monitored anesthesia care (MAC). Her main complaint at the moment is bleeding hemorrhoids. Her past history is relevant for hypertension, turbinate cancer (primary) which has been treated but she still gets occasionally epistaxis, hypothyroidism, noninsulin-dependent diabetes, and glaucoma. You see her in the preoperative area and place an IV and sedate her with 4 mg of midazolam. She is placed in a prone jackknife position on the operating table. You give her 50 μg of fentanyl and start a propofol infusion of 100 μg/kg/min. The surgeon uses a liberal amount of lidocaine and the surgery starts. Unfortunately, the procedure lasts longer than you have expected and it is now 1 h after the start and the patient is getting restless. You increase the propofol infusion, but to your dismay, you discover that the patient develops an upper airway obstruction. The oxygen saturation is falling. Things are not easy, as she is in the prone position. You turn the propofol off, place a facemask, and do a one-handed jaw thrust with one hand, while ventilating with the other hand. The oxygen saturation improves but only to 84%. You attempt to insert a Guedel airway but can't open her mouth.

Question

The options you have are waiting for the propofol to wear of, turning the patient supine, and maybe even placing an endotracheal tube in her trachea. However, is there anything else you can potentially do to improve the airway situations while the patient is prone?

J.G. Brock-Utne, *Case Studies of Near Misses in Clinical Anesthesia*,
DOI 10.1007/978-1-4419-1179-7_47,

Solution

This is a tricky question. Remember that the patient has a turbinate cancer and has occasionally epistaxis. Hence a nasal airway (nasal trumpet) is contraindicated.

In this case the patient slowly woke up from her propofol sedation and with that her airway obstruction cleared. Glycopyrrolate 0.6 mg and Ketamine 50 mg boluses were given IV successfully until the surgery was completed 25 min later.

Recommendation

Always remember the patient's comorbidities that may interfere or cause problems with your treatment. In this case, placing a nasal airway could have caused a major bleeding disaster.

Chapter 48
Case 48: Is the Patient Extubated?

You are called urgently to the ICU as the nurse can hear air escaping from the mouth of a 35-year-old morbidly obese patient. He is in the ICU recovering from a motor vehicle accident. When you arrive, his oxygen saturation is 84%, HR 110, and BP 130/90. You can easily hear the air escaping from his mouth. The nurse tells you that his oxygen saturation was, until a few minutes ago, 96% on FiO_2 of 100%. His face is severely swollen and he has large, thick neck with a diameter over 70 cm. The latter has been shown to indicate a difficult endotracheal intubation [1]. As you are about to let the pilot balloon down to advance the ETT further into the trachea, you discover that the pilot balloon is totally collapsed. You now discover that it will not inflate as it has a hole in it. You are reluctant to change the existing ETT with a tube changer as this may take too much time. Delaying the change of ETT could lead to a dramatic fall in oxygen saturation, with potentially disastrous consequences.

Question

You pack his throat with a 2 in. moist vaginal pack, to seal the glottic inlet and get his oxygen saturation up. This is however only a temporary measure, what else can you suggest?

J.G. Brock-Utne, *Case Studies of Near Misses in Clinical Anesthesia*,
DOI 10.1007/978-1-4419-1179-7_48,

Solution

Insert a Pilot Tube Repair Kit (BE409) (Metropolitan Medical Inc., Winchester, VA 22603). The needle, belonging to the Kit, is rubbed with an alcohol swab (Kendall Webcol, Alcohol prep. Mansfield, MA 02048). This is done to make the insertion of the needle easier after the pilot tubing have been cut away.

Causes of cuff leaks include small size ETT, torn cuff, faulty pilot balloon, and partial extubation. Recognition of partial extubation is critical as hypoxia, lost control of the airway, and death may occur. A pilot balloon can start to leak at any time, but it is not common. A study in the 115 ICU patients with cuff leaks found that 86% had a displaced ETT and 46% had the ETT tip located in the pharynx [2].

Recommendation

Always remember you can use the Pilot Tube Repair Kit to repair a leaking/non-functioning endotracheal cuff. This is especially true when you think it is unwise to replace a damaged ETT that is correctly placed in the trachea.

References

1. Brodsky JB, Lemmens HJM, Brock-Utne JG, Vierra M, Saidman IJ. Morbid obesity and tracheal intubation. Anesth Analg. 2002;94:732–6.
2. Mort TC. ETT cuff leak. A safety strategy. Crit Care Med. 2005;33(12):A85.

Chapter 49
Case 49: A Leaking Anesthesia Machine

You are scheduled to anesthetize a 45-year-old male (150 kg, 5 ft 10 in.) for cervical laminectomy. His medical history is significant for hypertension and noninsulin-dependent diabetes. On examination he complains about a stiff and painful neck when he moves it. You place an IV and sedate him with midazolam and take him to the operating room. In the operating room you place routine monitors and induce anesthesia. He is an easy mask and because of his neck problem you use a trachlight (Laerdal Medical, Stavanger, Norway) with an endotracheal tube (ETT) attached. The ETT is placed in the trachea without any problems. End-tidal CO_2 is seen and bilateral air entry is heard. An esophageal stethoscope is placed and the patient is turned prone. After he is positioned prone, you notice that the end-tidal CO_2 is decreased from 38 to 30 mmHg. The Apollo machine (Drager Medical, 233542 Lubeck, Germany) is now indicating that you have a leak in the machine and/or the breathing system. You confirm bilateral air entry and normal breath sounds. You commence manual ventilation but the leak is still there.

Question

Besides turning the patient supine and starting again, what will you do?

DOI 10.1007/978-1-4419-1179-7_49,

Solution

You remove the esophageal stethoscope and the leak goes away. Since the esophageal stethoscope was placed just before the patient was turned, the leak was not noticed before after the patient was prone.

Recommendation

Always look at the bellows or your airway pressures or airway alarms after you have placed an esophageal stethoscope. You won't regret it.

Chapter 50
Case 50: A Most Important Lesson

A 56-year-old woman (72 kg, 5 ft 10 in.) is scheduled for laparoscopic hysterectomy. She is classified as an ASA 1 and has no allergies. Her only medication is vitamins. General anesthesia is induced in a routine manner. You have a grade 1 view on laryngoscopy and pass a #7 endotracheal tube (ETT) without any problem. The ETT cuff is inflated. There is mist in the ETT and you see end-tidal CO_2. You confirm bilateral air entry. The ETT is secured at 22 cm at the lip. A temperature probe is placed in the esophagus and an upper body Bair Hugger is placed on the patient. The nurse inserts a urinary catheter. She hands you the urine catheter bag (Bard Criticore collection container, CR Bard Inc., Covington, GA 30014) and you place it in the Criticore (Fluid output and temperature monitor, CR Bard Inc., Covington, GA 30014). The surgeon has not come into the room. You are waiting for her to tell you what antibiotic she wants.

Suddenly you are aware of a change in the sound of the oxygen saturation monitor. You look up at the monitors and see that the oxygen saturation has fallen from 100 to 94% and is still falling. You note that there is no end-tidal CO_2, but you have a normal-looking airway wave form. Your noninvasive blood pressure machine is cycling.

Question

How will you deal with this problem?

J.G. Brock-Utne, *Case Studies of Near Misses in Clinical Anesthesia*,
DOI 10.1007/978-1-4419-1179-7_50, © Springer Science+Business Media, LLC 2011

Solution

One of the first things to do is to ascertain that you do have an adequate blood pressure. As mentioned, the first thing to do in these cases is to feel for the superficial temporal artery. If you feel a pulse there, then the systolic pressure is at least 60 mmHg. If no pulses are felt anywhere, then ACLS should be started.

In the above case, which landed in court, the anesthesiologist focused solely on the lack of end-tidal CO_2. Thinking that it was a capnograph malfunction, he called for a new capnograph. This delay caused a long delay in appropriate treatment of the hypotension and the patient became hypoxic and died 1 month later in the ICU.

Recommendation

Remember the monitors are only there to help you. If you are concerned that there is something wrong, then turn your attention to the patient. In other words, look and feel the patient. Remember what Hein said in 1965: "When technology is master, we will reach disaster faster."

Chapter 51
Case 51: Transsphenoidal Resection of a Pituitary Tumor

Today you are in the preoperative clinic. A 58-year-old lady (86 kg, 5 ft 9 in.) is scheduled next week for a transsphenoidal resection of a pituitary adenoma. She has a past history of coronary artery disease, hypertension, and an aortic valve replacement (mechanical prostheses). The latter was done 8 years ago. She is taking hypertensive medication and warfarin. She has no allergies and her last general anesthetic (aortic valve replacement) was uneventful. The neurosurgeon has included a note with the patient's chart. In that he wants you to outline the medical management of the anticoagulation therapy.

Questions

He wants to know:

1. When should the warfarin be stopped prior to surgery and when should it be resumed?
2. Do you recommend IV heparin or LMWH (enoxaparin) (Lovenox), as a bridging therapy just prior to and/or after the surgery? If so, when should that be stopped and when may it be resumed?

   What is your recommendation?

J.G. Brock-Utne, *Case Studies of Near Misses in Clinical Anesthesia*,
DOI 10.1007/978-1-4419-1179-7_51, © Springer Science+Business Media, LLC 2011

Solutions

I have unfortunately seen two patients with aortic valve mechanical replacements who both died postoperatively after transsphenoidal resections of pituitary adenomas. Both died within 36 h. One died because the anticoagulation was started too early (12 h after end of surgery) leading to uncontrollable surgical bleeding. The other died from starting the anticoagulation therapy too late (36 h after the end of surgery) leading to the clotting of the aortic valve. There is no clinical study to indicate the correct way to approach this problem. The best thing to do is to stop the warfarin 6–7 days preoperatively. When the INR becomes subtherapeutic, then you can start Lovenox 1 or 1.5 mg/kg (see packed insert for detailed instructions). Since the LMWH has a longer action than the standard unfractionated heparin, the LMWH must be stopped 12–24 h prior to surgery. The advantage of LMWH is that you do not have to check PTT before the day of surgery. With IV infusion of heparin, you must admit the patient and follow the PTT. Should the INR remain elevated (>1.5 IU) then oral vitamin K can be given (1–2.5 mg) but the INR needs to be checked prior to surgery.

Warfarin should be resumed as soon as possible on postoperative day 1 or 2. Bridging therapy can also be resumed and continued until therapeutic warfarin anticoagulation has been reached.

The real problem in these cases relates to when to restart the anticoagulation medication. Keeping the patient in the ICU with the arterial line or CVP line for hourly coagulation studies and checking for hemostasis is imperative in these cases.

Recommendation

These patients are at high risk for either uncontrollable postoperative surgical bleeding or clotting of their aortic valves. Getting surgical homeostasis and the anticoagulation right, both before and after the operation, is imperative for a good outcome.

Chapter 52
Case 52: Spinal Reconstruction and Fusion in a Chronic Pain Patient

The surgeon has started closing after 4.5 h of lumbar spinal reconstruction and fusion. The patient is a 45-year-old man (90 kg, 5 ft 11 in.) who is lying prone on a Wilson frame. His head is in a Prone View (Dupaco, Union City, CA 94587). He is undergoing this surgery because of chronic pain to his back and difficulty in walking following a motor vehicle accident 2 years ago. He is on chronic pain medication that includes methadone, gabapentin, and a fentanyl patch. He is otherwise healthy. The anesthetic maintenance has been nitrous oxide in oxygen with isoflurane. You are concerned that he will be aware of pain during the procedure so you have been giving him narcotics titrated to his vital signs. Throughout the course of the operation, he has received a total of fentanyl 500 μg, dilaudid 2 mg, and morphine 20 mg. In the last half an hour, he has also received 50 mg of meperidine 30 mg of ketamine IV. Ten minutes from the end, you turn off the isoflurane and leave him on nitrous oxide and oxygen. You still have not reversed his neuromuscular blockade. His vital signs just as you are about to turn him are HR 82 bpm, BP 130/85. These values seem to indicate to you that he is adequately anesthetized and analgesic. Of course you can't be sure.

Question

Besides checking his oxygenation, HR and BP, what is the first thing you should do after turning the patient supine, to ascertain if the patient is adequately anesthetized and/or analgesic?

J.G. Brock-Utne, *Case Studies of Near Misses in Clinical Anesthesia*,
DOI 10.1007/978-1-4419-1179-7_52, © Springer Science+Business Media, LLC 2011

Solution

Look at the pupils. If they are widely dilated you know that the patient has not been given sufficient analgesics. If this happened to me, I would give after the patient is turned a lot of IV narcotics. I titrate the amount I give to the patient's respiratory rate between 8 and 12. When the patient has pain, the rate will be high. I find meperidine to be the easiest drug to use in these cases. I don't however give more than 2 mg/kg. If I need more narcotics then I change to morphine or dilaudid. It is most rewarding to have a chronic pain patient arriving in the recovery room with NO pain.

I am grateful to Dr. Merlin Larson of UCSF, Department of Anesthesia, for providing the table entitled "Pupillary abnormalities noted during the surgical anesthesia" (Table 52.1).

I see some of my colleagues reverse the neuromuscular blockade prior to placing the patient supine. I don't do that. If you do reverse the blockade prior to turning, then the patient can move and trash about and potentially injure themselves. The surgeon is also not impressed. He will prefer you to take your time and wake the patient, in these cases, up slowly. I always give the reversal after the patient is turned.

Recommendation

In chronic pain patient undergoing surgery in the supine position, it is easy to evaluate if the patient has adequate analgesia by looking at the pupils. In the prone position where there is no readily access to the pupils, it is difficult. Hence, in the prone chronic patient, it is imperative to look at the pupils as soon as you can after the patient is placed on the supine position.

Table 52.1 Pupillary abnormalities noted during the surgical anesthesia

	Affected pupil size	Direct light reaction	Consensual reaction of affected pupil	Consensual reaction of unaffected pupil
Pharmacologic causes				
Topical Epinephrine or Phenylephrine	Large	Absent or sluggish[a]	Absent or sluggish[a]	Normal
Topical Atropine or Scopolamine	Large	Absent	Absent	Normal
Local anesthetics injected into orbit	Large	Absent	Absent	Normal if only oculomotor nerve is blocked
Local anesthetics injected into the orbit	Large	Absent	Absent	Absent if both oculomotor and optic nerves are blocked
Structural lesions				
Optic nerve trauma during endoscopic surgery	Normal – no anisocoria	Absent	Normal	Absent
Oculomotor nerve trauma during endoscopic surgery	Large	Absent	Absent	Normal
Oculomotor and optic nerve trauma during endoscopic surgery	Large	Absent	Absent	Absent
Acute trauma or paralysis of dilator sympathetic fibers (acute Horner's)	Normal – no anisocoria[b]	Present[a]	Present[a]	Present[b]
Third nerve compression (uncus, aneurysm)	Large	Absent	Absent	Present or sluggish[c]

Pupillary abnormalities noted during the surgical anesthesia. Exam of pupil size and reactivity, both direct and consensual, can greatly help in identifying an etiology for the pupil abnormality. Courtesy of Mark D. Rollins, MD, Swetha Pakala, MD, and Merlin D. Larson, MD

[a] Anesthetized patients usually have small (miotic) pupils because of concurrent opioid administration. The light reflex in miotic pupils can be difficult to appreciate visually and pupillometric devices may be required to document the presence or absence of a light reflex

[b] The dilator muscle has no sympathetic tone in anesthetized subjects, so the anisocoria of Horner's syndrome is not present during anesthesia

[c] A historical analysis of the case is essential when considering this diagnosis. Lacking recent head trauma or a patient undergoing a neurosurgical procedure, there are no case reports of intracranial hemorrhage producing new onset of anisocoria during general anesthesia

Chapter 53
Case 53: A Repeat Back Operation in a Patient Who Has Had Postoperative Visual Loss in the Past

You are in the preoperative clinic. The nurse asks your opinion about a 65-year-old man (85 kg, 5 ft 9 in.) who is scheduled for a repeat one level lumbosacral laminectomy. Two years ago after a back operation, he developed temporary bilateral postoperative visual loss (POVL). He was seen by an ophthalmologist at that time, who diagnosed ischemic optic neuropathy [1–3]. The patient is obviously very concerned about the upcoming surgery, but tells you that he cannot live with the back pain and would rather take his chances. The operation will take 1–2 h. The patient has a history of type 2 diabetes mellitus, hypertension, and is a smoker. He takes glyburide and captopril.

He asks you: Is there anything that can be done to attempt to prevent this from happening again?

You tell him that he has a lot of risk factors for POVL. These include diabetes, hypertension, obesity, smoking, arterioscleroses, and an age above 50. On the positive side, there should be minimal blood loss, he does not have narrow angle glaucoma or sickle cell anemia, renal failure, GI ulcers, polycythemia vera, and collagen vascular disorders.

Question

Is there anything you would suggest that the anesthesiologist do prior to the operation to attempt to minimize/prevent POVL?

J.G. Brock-Utne, *Case Studies of Near Misses in Clinical Anesthesia*,
DOI 10.1007/978-1-4419-1179-7_53,

Solutions

Intraocular pressure (IOP) increase is thought to be a major contributor to POVL. Cheng et al. [4] has shown that IOP significantly increased in prone anesthetized patients compared to supine anesthetized patients. An increase in IOP leads to a decrease in ocular perfusion pressure [5]. It has been proposed that giving prophylactically a cardiac selective betablocker like Betaxolol eyedrops to patients who are undergoing back surgery may be beneficial in preventing POVL [6]. Another study has suggested a 15° elevation in the prone position which was effective in reducing IOP in anesthetized patients and the effect was apparent after 3 h [7].

In a retrospective study [8], it was suggested that intraoperative risk factors do develop POVL, like length of time in the prone position, IV fluids >8 L, hypothermia <35°C, blood pressure below 20% of baseline, and postoperative facial edema were more important than preoperative patient factors.

A good article to read is one by Warner [9]. It deals with a medical plaintiff's expert opinion in cases of postoperative blindness.

For those interested in studying this problem, Grant et al. [10] have suggested a clinically practical method for measuring the IOP, ocular perfusion pressure, and the ocular perfusion in prone patients. They suggested using a combination of the Proneview Helmet system (Dupaco, Oceanside, CA) and a Jackson spine table (Orthopedic systems, Inc., Union City, CA).

Recommendation

POVL is a rare but serious complication related to prone position surgery. Eliminating risk factors, like elevation of the head during the operation and possibly the use of prophylactic Betaxolol eyedrops, may have some beneficial effects.

References

1. Williams EL, Hart WM, Tempelhoff R. Postoperative ischemic optic neuropathy. Anesth Analg. 1995;80:1018–29.
2. Tempelhoff R. An optic nerve at risk and a prolonged surgery in the prone position. Anesthesiology. 2008;108:775–6.
3. Shen Y, Drum M, Roth S. The prevalence of perioperative visual loss in the United States: a 10 year study from 1996 to 2005 of spinal, orthopedic, cardiac and general surgery. Anesth Analg. 2009;109:1534–45.
4. Cheng MA, Todorov A, Tempelhoff R, McHugh T, Crourder CM, Lauryssen C. The effect of prone position on intraocular pressure in anesthetized patients. Anesthesiology. 2001;95:1351–5.
5. Hayreh SS. Anterior ischemic optic neuropathy. Clin Neurosci. 1997;4:251–63.
6. Brock-Utne JG. Submitted research project at Stanford University medical center.

7. Fukui K, Ahmad M, McHugh T, Tempelhoff R, Cheng MA. The effect of head elevation on intraocular pressure in anesthetized patients undergoing prone position spine surgery. Anesthesiology. 2004:A 382 (Abstract).
8. Dulitz M, Wong C. Postoperative visual loss. A retrospective chart review. Anesthesiology. 2004:A 1286 (Abstracts).
9. Warner MA. Postoperative visual loss. Experts, data and practice. Anesthesiology. 2006;105:641–2.
10. Grant GP, Turbin RE, Bennett HL, Szirth BC, Heary RF. Use of the Proneview Helmet system with a modified table platform for open access to the eyes during prone spine surgery. Anesth Analg. 2006;103:499–500.

Chapter 54
Case 54: Respiratory Arrest in the Recovery Room

You are scheduled to anesthetize a 9-year-old boy (12 kg) for a right hernia repair. His past medical history is unremarkable. He has been healthy all his life up to this point. He has no allergies and the family history is negative for anesthesia-related problems. You examine the child and find nothing abnormal. He has got an IV (20 gauge) in the back of his right hand. This has been placed by a pediatrician for preoperative antibiotics. Since the IV is working, you sedate him with 0.5 mg of midazolam IV. In the operating room, routine monitors are placed. You induce anesthesia with propofol. The patient falls asleep and is an easy mask. You ventilate him with sevoflurane 1–3% in 100% oxygen. Through the IV you give 4 mg of vecuronium. After 3 min you check with your nerve stimulator and discover that the patient is not adequately relaxed. You check the IV and find it now nonfunctioning. A new IV is inserted and a repeat dose of 4 mg of vecuronium is given. Within 3 min, the nerve stimulator indicates that the patient is adequately relaxed. An endotracheal tube (ETT) is inserted atraumatically into the trachea. Routine anesthesia is instituted with nitrous oxide 70% in oxygen with sevoflurane and meperidine 15 mg. The surgery commences and concludes uneventfully. At the end of the anesthetic you reverse the neuromuscular blockade, spontaneous ventilation, and the ETT is removed. The child is taken to the recovery room asleep but arousable.

Fifteen minutes later you are called to the recovery room. You are told that the boy is not breathing and oxygen saturation is now 76%. You tell the nurse to start artificial ventilation and run to the recovery room. In the recovery room, the nurse is successfully ventilating the child and the oxygen saturation is now 98% and his vital signs are HR of 135 bpm and a BP of 80/45.

J.G. Brock-Utne, *Case Studies of Near Misses in Clinical Anesthesia*,
DOI 10.1007/978-1-4419-1179-7_54, © Springer Science+Business Media, LLC 2011

Questions

What will you do? What can the cause of this dilemma be?

Solution

You quickly insert an ETT into the trachea. Oxygenation and his vital signs are normal. You wonder what happened when you see that the IV that had failed you in the operating room now seems to be working. The nurse informs you, with some sense of achievement, that she has managed to get the IV to work. You call for a nerve stimulator and confirm that the patient is completely relaxed. You realize that the cause of the respiratory failure was most likely the vecuronium that remained in the original IV. The drug entered the systemic circulation when the nurse got it working again in the recovery room.

An intraoperative nonfunctioning IV is not an uncommon problem. The above case is unusual, but when the IV is hidden from view, infiltration can occur. I have seen a case of a 60-year-old man who had his left arm amputated above the elbow after a 4-h routine coronary artery bypass operation because of excessive IV infiltration. We have also described a hidden IV unintentionally severed by a surgeon [1]. This could have led to a near disaster. If I cannot see the IV catheter entering the vein, I will not use it unless absolutely necessary. If I must use it, I check it regularly for patency.

Recommendation

If an IV is not working properly, remove it immediately. This should prevent potentially serious disasters.

Reference

1. Kim A, Brock-Utne JG. Another potential problem with the "hidden IV". Can J Anaesth. 1998;45:495–6.

Chapter 55
Case 55: Bispectral Index – What Does It Mean?

Today you are anesthetizing a 70-year-old woman scheduled for repair of an internal iliac aneurysm. She has Type-2 diabetes mellitus, hypertension, and stable angina. The latter is treated medically. She takes metformin (500 mg bid), glibenclamide (2.5 mg/day), metoprolol (25 mg bid), aspirin (100 mg/day), and atorvastatin (20 mg/day). Her blood sugar is 250 mg/100 mL. As requested she has not taken her oral hypoglycemic on the day of surgery. You see her in the preoperative area and tell her that you will be using the Bispectral Index Scale (BIS) (Aspect Medical Systems, Natick, MA) to assess her depth of anesthesia. Since this is the first time you are using the BIS monitor, you have a BIS monitor representative present in the operating room during the procedure. You introduce her to him and she consents that he may be present. On the way to the operating room, you sedate her with 2 mg of midazolam.

In the operating room, you place the BIS monitor on the patient (A-2000 XP monitor, Aspect MS, Natick, MA) and activate its continuous mode. Thereafter the patient is anesthetized with fentanyl 100 μg, propofol 120 mg, and 40 mg of rocuronium. When the patient is adequately anesthetized and relaxed, you secure the airway with an endotracheal tube (ETT). Anesthesia is maintained with oxygen in air and sevoflurane set for an end-tidal value of 1.1%. The BIS is now at 38–46. You place an arterial line and send off a blood gas. The surgery commences. About 15 min later, the blood gas is shown to be normal. But you do note that her blood sugar is now 280 mg/100 mL. Six international unit of purified human neutral insulin is given. After about 10 min the BIS value decreases and settles to 12–16. Since you have never used the BIS before, you ask the representative if he can explain this sudden decrease in BIS value. You have given no other drugs except the insulin and there are no adverse surgical events. There are no changes in hemodynamic parameters. Furthermore, you have not changed the ventilation or the sevoflurane concentration.

The representative says the lower BIS number means that the patient is deeply anesthetized. He suggests that you decrease your anesthetic. You are not sure what

J.G. Brock-Utne, *Case Studies of Near Misses in Clinical Anesthesia*,
DOI 10.1007/978-1-4419-1179-7_55, © Springer Science+Business Media, LLC 2011

to think as your experience tells you that the patient is adequately anesthetized. You are also unsure if the BIS monitor can assess the depth of anesthesia. You look at the patient's pupils and they are nicely constricted. There is no sweating of the head and hands. In your opinion, the patient is adequately anesthetized and you are reluctant to change anything.

Question

Will you lighten the anesthetic or will you ask the representative to take his machine and leave or what will you do?

Solution

You go online on the operating room computer. Here you find two references that severe hypoglycemia may induce a decrease in electroencephalogram in both diabetic and nondiabetic patients [1–3]. In the case report [3] to which this case refers, a finger stick informs you that the patient has severe hypoglycemia. You correct it and the BIS increased to 35–39 over 4–8 min. A rapid change in BIS with correction of hypoglycemia has been reported in a patient in an ICU [4].

The BIS has been marketed as an EEG-based monitor of anesthetic effect and thereby decreasing awareness during anesthesia. However, BIS has severe limitations as a monitor to measure the depth of anesthesia. The BIS is calculated based on the correlation between the phases of the different wave components of the EEG with 0 meaning no EEG activity and 100 fully awake. The effect of different anesthetic agents on the BIS value is dependent on the drugs used. Propofol, midazolam, and isoflurane decrease the BIS to 40–60 and this number is believed (no proof) to indicate a level suitable for general anesthesia [4]. Unfortunately, when a combination of different anesthetics is used (the most common occurrence), the interpretation of the BIS level is not as straightforward. When opioids are administered concurrently with propofol for induction of anesthesia, patients lose consciousness at higher BIS levels than when propofol is given alone [5, 6]. It is interesting to note that the addition of nitrous oxide and ketamine results in a deeper level of anesthesia, but the BIS level actually increases. BIS levels may also be affected by changes in degree of neuromuscular blockade during anesthesia and surgery because of electromyographic (EMG) activity. An increase in EMG activity may increase the BIS value as may the use of succinylcholine.

In the first and only large-scale study to document the incidence of awareness, when BIS is used, has shown no benefit of the BIS to prevent awareness [7]. In the study 13 patients, despite BIS monitoring, had awareness. Roughly, 40% of their patients were monitored with the BIS. It is telling that the BIS-monitored group had a HIGHER incidence of awareness (0.18%) than the control group (0.1%). The authors [6] state that this trend was not statistically significant without quoting any statistical analyses. However, McCulloch [8] states that when he analyzes the data given in their table 6, a p value of 0.17 is seen.

In the above case report [3], it is interesting to note that when the hypoglycemia was corrected, the BIS went back to its preinsulin injection level.

Recommendation

The clinician must know BIS's limitations and be aware that it will not help contribute to the prevention of awareness.

References

1. Gilbert TT, Wagner MR, Halukurike V, Paz HI, Garland A. Use of Bispectral electroencephalogram monitoring to assess neurologic status in unsedated critical ill patients. Crit Care Med. 2001;29:1996–2000.
2. Pramming S, Thorsteinsson B, Stigsby B, Binder C. Glycaemic threshold changes in electroencephalograms during hypoglycemia in patients with insulin dependent diabetes. BMJ. 1988;296:665–7.
3. Naryanaswamy M. Decrease in Bispectral index while correcting hyperglycemia and increase in Bispectral index with correction of hypoglycemia. Anesth Analg. 2009;109:995.
4. Vivien B, Olivier Langeron O, Bruno Riou B. Increase in bispectral index (BIS) while correcting a severe hypoglycemia. Anesth Analg. 2002;95:1824–5.
5. Glass PS, Bloom M, Kearse L, Rosow C, Sebel P, Manberg P. Bispectral analysis measured sedatin and memory effects of propofol, midazolam, isoflurane and alfentanil in healthy volunteers. Anesthesiology. 1997;86:836–47.
6. Lysakowski C, Dumont L, Pellegrini M, Clergue F, Tassonyi E. Effect of fentany, alfentanil, remifentanil and sufentanil on loss of consciousness and Bispectral Index during propofol induction of anaesthesia. Br J Anaesth. 2001;86:523–7.
7. Sebel PS, Bowdle TA, Ghoneim MM, Rampil IJ, Padilla RE, Gan TJ, et al. The incidence of awareness during anesthesia: a multicenter United States study. Anesth Analg. 2004;99:833–9.
8. McCulloch TJ. Use of BIS monitoring was not associated with a reduced incidence of awareness. Anesth Analg. 2004;100:1221–2.

Chapter 56
Case 56: Neonatal Laparoscopic Surgery

It is midnight and you are on call. A 1-day-old male (36 week gestation) is scheduled for laparoscopic repair of Duodenal Atresia. He was delivered uneventfully a few hours ago. He weighs 2 kg and his history, physical exam, and laboratory results are unremarkable. You see him in the NICU and notice fresh blood at the stump of the umbilical vein. You are told that an attempt at umbilical vein cannulation failed. There is no umbilical clamp but a tie has been placed around the umbilical stump instead. The patient has a working peripheral IV. In the operating room, standard monitoring is placed on the child. The child is preoxygenated and a rapid-sequence technique with propofol, rocuronium, and cricoids pressure ensues. His airway was secured with 3.0 endotracheal tube (ETT). Anesthesia is maintained with sevoflurane in oxygen and air. Another peripheral IV is placed and fentanyl 1 μg/kg is given IV. Surgery starts with the insertion of the umbilical trocar. Suddenly, you notice that the end-tidal CO_2 decreases from 28 to 6 mmHg. There is no recordable oxygen saturation, the noninvasive blood pressure machine is cycling, and the heart rate decreases from 140 to 100 bpm. There are no pulses to be palpated. The noninvasive BP gives you a reading of 40/20 and the HR is 96 on the EKG. You discontinue the sevoflurane and start ventilating with 100% oxygen.

You look to the surgeons for a possible CO_2 embolism, but they have not started insufflating the peritoneal cavity with CO_2. The surgeons exclude intra-abdominal trauma caused by the trocar by partially insufflating the peritoneal cavity and discovering no active bleeding. There is no pneumothorax based on your clinical exam. You examine your IV lines for evidence of air. There is none and you know you have been very careful not to introduce any air when you put your line in. In the absence of a diagnosis, you commence cardiopulmonary resuscitation (CPR).

J.G. Brock-Utne, *Case Studies of Near Misses in Clinical Anesthesia*,
DOI 10.1007/978-1-4419-1179-7_56,

Question

What can the problem be, as you have excluded CO_2 embolism, air embolism from your IV line, hypovolemia caused by the surgeon, and a pneumothorax? Furthermore, you don't believe this is an anaphylactic reaction.

Solution

Air embolus, not from the IV line, but from the umbilical vein was the cause of the cardiovascular collapse in this neonate. This is similar to the case reported by Lalwani and Aliason [1]. As the surgeon withdrew the trocar and CPR started, they noticed active bleeding from the umbilical vein stump. The stump was ligated and the abdomen closed. An echocardiography demonstrated large amounts of air in the right ventricle, pulmonary arteries, and aorta. After 10 min of CPR and epinephrine in the Trendelenburg position, end-tidal CO_2 reappeared, the pulses became palpable, and there was a pulse oximeter wave form. The child was taken to the ICU and ventilated overnight. He made an uneventful recovery and was discharged home 10 days later. At 1 month, he was developing normally [1].

Although not mentioned in the case report referred to above [1], it is most likely that an attempt at umbilical vein cannulation was done shortly after delivery. Therefore, the umbilical clamp could have been removed or never placed. In lieu of a clamp a tie was placed, but the latter not sufficient to prevent bleeding or entrainment of air.

The cause of the dilemma, as mentioned, was an air embolus. This could have been caused by the trocar injuring the umbilical vein prior to peritoneal insufflation. Another reason could be the failed umbilical vein cannulation, prior to the surgery, led to a leaking umbilical vein. Also the incorrectly applied tie to the umbilical cord most likely further contributed to the leak. After the induction of general anesthesia, with ensuing vasodilation and a drop in central venous pressure – venous air entrainment occurred.

Recommendation

Fresh blood seen from the umbilical stump, with or without a clamp or a tie, must always be taken seriously.

Reference

1. Lalwani K, Aliason I. Cardiac arrest in the neonate during laprascopic surgery. Anesth Analg. 2009;109:760–2.

Chapter 57
Case 57: Total IV Anesthesia

Today you are anesthetizing a 49-year-old female (48 kg, 5 ft 6 in.) for a laparoscopic cholecystectomy. Her past history is significant for a cardiac arrest under general anesthesia 25 years before. No other information is available, but she tells you that there is a family history of malignant hyperthermia. She has undergone more than ten surgical procedures under general anesthesia without any problems. The last one was for a knee replacement 8 months ago. There is no information available as to the anesthetic techniques used in all these case. She has no allergies and is otherwise healthy. Her laboratory values are within normal limits. With the history of malignant hyperthermia, you decide on a nontriggering anesthetic using a total intravenous anesthetic technique. You place a 20-gauge IV catheter in her left hand, sedate her with 4 mg of midazolam IV, and take her to the operating room. Here you place routine monitors and induce general anesthesia with fentanyl, propofol, and vecuronium. An endotracheal tube (ETT) is placed uneventfully into her trachea. She is ventilated with air in 50% oxygen. You place a BIS monitor, although you have not much confident in this monitor (see Chap. 55). But since the monitor is available, you decide to use it. The surgeon insists that the arms are tucked along her body. After that is done you make sure the IV is working. Anesthetic maintained is with propofol 100 μg/kg/min with remifentanil 0.09 μg/kg/min. The surgeon is known to be slow, so you expect this procedure to last about 2 h.

Questions

Is there anything else you would have done prior to the surgery? Or are you happy for the surgeon to start?

J.G. Brock-Utne, *Case Studies of Near Misses in Clinical Anesthesia*,
DOI 10.1007/978-1-4419-1179-7_57, © Springer Science+Business Media, LLC 2011

Solution

Put in another IV. Ideally when you are giving a total IV anesthetic, you should have two IVs, one for fluid infusion and one for infusion of the anesthetic mixture. Furthermore, it is vital to be able to see the IVs at all times. The surgeon should be informed about your concerns and needs and should try to accommodate you.

For the IV that is used solely for the maintenance of anesthesia, I use the Mini Bifuse 2 to 1 administration set (Smiths Medical, Brisbane QLD 4113). This is ideal as it gives both remifentanil and propofol through different ports, close to the IV insertion site. The dead space for the drug infusion is therefore minimal.

When I do a total IV anesthetic, I always have two IVs. A case of awareness during surgery has been recorded in the literature [1]. In that case a total IV anesthetic was given through one IV. The intravenous catheter malfunctioned and the IV anesthetic stopped flowing. The anesthesiologist was alerted to the problem by a sudden increase in heart rate. The patient developed posttraumatic stress disorder (PTSD), which took months to heal. It is unclear if this patient had awareness with pain or without pain [1].

Recommendation

When using a total IV anesthetic technique, two IVs are essential. One IV is used to give the anesthetic and the other for IV fluids etc.

Reference

1. Mashour GA, Wang LYJ, Esaki RK, Naughton NN. Operating room desensitization as a novel treatment for post-traumatic stress disorder after intraoperative awareness. Anesthesiology. 2008;109:927–8.

Chapter 58
Case 58: An ICU Patient

A 58-year-old male is admitted from a medical ward to the ICU. He has had a severe GI bleed. On examination he is confused, hypoxic, tachycardiac, and hypotensive. His past history is significant for cirrhosis and renal insufficiency. His left arm is seen to be full of eccymosis, edema, and is extremely tender. There is significant erythema around an 18-G IV on the back of his left hand. This is the only IV he has. It is also the only IV that has been used since admission, 48 h ago, for resuscitation and blood products. You remove the 18-G IV and ask for a stat surgical consult for the left arm.

You place an internal jugular central venous access line and a right radial arterial line and aggressively start treatment for septic shock. This includes fluids, antibiotics, and pressors. A blood gas tells you the patient is in respiratory failure ($paO_2 < 60$ mm Hg:and/ or $paCO_2 > 55$ mm Hg). The patient is placed on mechanical ventilation via an endotracheal tube. A surgeon arrives and diagnoses the arm as having a necrotizing soft-tissue infection. One hour later, the patient is taken to the operating room for urgent extensive surgical debridement. The blood and tissue cultures are both later positive for *Escherichia coli*.

Twenty-four hours later, the patient is hemodynamically stable and weaned off pressures. However, he has a significant opiate requirement due to the pain in his left arm. You call in the hospital's acute pain team. Unfortunately, they are only partly successful in decreasing the pain with a combination of diluted PCA, ketamine, and a fentanyl patch.

Despite the poor pain control, you attempt to wean the patient from the ventilator over the next 4 days. However, every trial fails, due to hypoxia and/or apnea.

J.G. Brock-Utne, *Case Studies of Near Misses in Clinical Anesthesia*,
DOI 10.1007/978-1-4419-1179-7_58,

Question

Is there anything you would suggest to control the pain better and get the patient weaned from the ventilator?

Solution

A supraclavicular nerve catheter provided immediate pain relief. Opiates etc. were discontinued and the patient was successfully extubated. The next day he was transferred out of the ICU back to the medical ward. His pain was managed via catheter infusion of local anesthetic for 3 days (Hansen JA and Lin LH, 2009, personal communication).

By using a continuous nerve catheter, to block the brachial plexus, the patient's ICU stay was shortened and his recovery speedier.

Recommendation

ICU patients, with multisystem dysfunction and concomitant necrotizing soft-tissue limb infection, may benefit from a regional block. The patient coagulation status must be checked prior to the block.

Chapter 59
Case 59: A New Onset of Atrial Fibrillation in the Recovery Room

You have anesthetized a 68-year-old female (62 kg, 5 ft 8 in.) for an inguinal hernia repair. Her past history was significant for a 30-year smoking history, hypertension, noninsulin-dependent diabetes mellitus, and hyperlipidemia. There had been no past history of cardiac arrhythmias. The preoperative EKG was normal. The patient and her daughter were very nervous about the general anesthetic, but the patient refused a monitored anesthetic care plan (IV sedation and the liberal use of local anesthetic by the surgeon). The patient has never had a general anesthetic or surgical procedure before. After placing the IV in her left hand, you sedate her with midazolam up to 4 mg. The general anesthetic with an LMA was uneventful. The operation lasted for 70 min and she was given 2 L of IV crystalloids. Her vital signs remained stable throughout. The urine output was not measured and the blood loss was less than 100 mL.

In the recovery room, you give the recovery room nurse your report. As you stand by the bedside, you notice the patient's EKG is now showing a new onset of rapid atrial fibrillation (AF). The patient has no complain of breathlessness or chest pain. She appears comfortable. The heart rate is 130 bpm, BP 130/80. She is on 3 L of oxygen via a nasal cannula. The oxygen saturation is 96%. You order a stat 12 lead. This confirms the diagnosis of AF.

You call the surgeon. He looks at the patient and EKG and says: "What is the problem?" You explain that the patient has had a new onset of AF and should be admitted to a monitored bed and treated by a cardiologist. The surgeon does not agree and suggest that as soon as the patient has met the recovery room discharge criteria, she should go home and be seen by her cardiologist the next day. You object, but he is adamant.

J.G. Brock-Utne, *Case Studies of Near Misses in Clinical Anesthesia*,
DOI 10.1007/978-1-4419-1179-7_59,

Question

What will you do?

Solution

This happened to a friend of mine within a week of starting his new job.

My friend spoke to the daughter and diplomatically explained what had happened and what you wanted to do. You inform her of the following options:

1. Tell the surgeon to admit her mother to a monitored bed and to be treated by a cardiologist (this is in your opinion the best).
2. Do as the surgeon suggested.
3. Do as the surgeon suggest but take her straight to the nearest emergency room.
4. Attempt to treat her in the recovery room but failing that she must be admitted.

My friend was asked by the daughter to attempt #4. Since the patient was in the recovery room, the patient was under my friend's care. He gave her IV diltiazem 15 mg over a 15-min period. The ventricular response promptly decreased to 70–75 bpm. The BP was 149/75 and a new 12-lead EKG showed a normal sinus rhythm with no evidence of ischemia. The daughter elected to take the mother home as she was worried about the added stress to her mother of admission to a monitored bed. The next day the daughter took her mother to the cardiologist. Six months later, the mother's heart was still in normal sinus rhythm.

Recommendations

1. A new onset of AF should never be ignored. If in the recovery room the AF cannot be corrected to sinus rhythm, then an urgent cardiology consultation is sought in the recovery room. Thereafter, admission to a monitored bed is the only correct treatment option.
2. When health providers differ in their opinions as to treatment, it is imperative to inform the patient/relatives of their options. Also it is essential to record in the chart what was told, agreed upon, and treatment given. Informing the patient and relatives as to what their options are is imperative. Also writing down everything in the chart, as to what was done and what was agreed upon, is essential. These cases can stretch your diplomatic talents way beyond what you were taught in medical school.

Chapter 60
Case 60: A Rapid Increase in Core Body Temperature

You are scheduled to anesthetize a 53-year-old female (130 kg, 5 ft 9 in.) for a laparoscopic revision of a gastric bypass and hiatal hernia. Two years before she had a laparoscopic Roux-en-Y gastric bypass. Her past medical history is significant for hypertension and morbid obesity. She reported no problems with her previous anesthetics. There are no allergies. A routine general anesthetic consisting of midazolam, fentanyl, propofol, and succinylcholine and an endotracheal tube placement is uneventful. Maintenance of anesthesia is with N_2O in oxygen with sevoflurane and vecuronium. An orogastric tube, an esophageal temperature probe, and an upper body Bair Hugger (42°C) are placed.

The operation starts. Approximately 30 min later, the temperature increases to a peak of 38.8°C from 36.2°C. The heart rate, BP, and most importantly the end-tidal CO_2 remain unchanged.

Questions

You are at a loss to understand what is happening. What will you do? Are you or should you be concerned?

DOI 10.1007/978-1-4419-1179-7_60,

Solution

You place another temperature probe (Liquid Crystal temperature indicator) on the forehead and another temperature probe just in the back of pharynx and find them both reading 36°C. You now pull the esophageal temperature probe back and discover that the temperature falls. The cause of this dilemma was the use of cautery adjacent to the temperature sensor during the dissection of the esophagus [1]. This problem has also been reported during laparoscopic Nissen fundoplication in a pediatric patient [2]. A hot lamp over a neonate can also give a faulty increase in temperature [3].

Recommendation

When there is a rapid rise in a patient's temperature, as recorded from one measuring site, check the patient's temperature from other sites.

References

1. Egan BJ, Clark C. A spurious increase of core temperature during laparoscopy. Anesth Analg. 2009;108:677.
2. Sanders JC. Deep positioning of an esophageal temperature probe may lead to overestimation of core body temperature during laparascopic Nissen fundoplication in infants. Paediatr Anaesth. 2005;15:351–2.
3. Claure RE, Brock-Utne JG. Liquid crystal temperature indicator – a potential serious problem in pediatric anesthesia. Can J Anaesth. 1998;45:828.

Chapter 61
Case 61: Prolonged Surgery

You are called to the ER to evaluate a 54-year-old man (80 kg, 6 ft 2 in.) who has sustained a right acetabular fracture after falling off his motorbike. He is booked for an open reduction and internal fixation. His past medical history is significant for a 35-year-old smoking history. He has no allergies. The physical exam reveals no other injuries. He denies any loss of consciousness at the time of his fall and he claims he remembers everything.

In the operating room, a rapid sequence induction with thiopental and succinylcholine is induced. The airway is secured with an endotracheal tube in his trachea. A right radial artery line is placed. The patient is placed in the left lateral position. The left arm is pronated and placed on an armboard and supported by foam so that the elbow is bent to an angle of >60°. The right arm is placed on an airplane splint. Both arms are <90° to the operating table, padded and secured.

Maintenance of anesthesia is with N_2O in oxygen, sevoflurane, fentanyl, and morphine. The operation lasts for 7 h. Blood loss exceeds 7 L. This is replaced with packs of red blood cells, albumin, hespan, and crystalloids. During the operation, many arterial blood gases are sent to the laboratory and all are within normal limits. At the conclusion of the surgery, the HCT is 30. The patient has been hemodynamically stable throughout. He is taken to the recovery room, awake, pain free, extubated, and breathing spontaneously.

On postoperative day 1, the patient complains of weakness in his left hand. On examination the left hand and forearm are edematous (+1). There is no sensory deficit. However, wrist extension and flexion, finger extension and flexion, and finger abduction and adduction are weak at 1/5. The right arm is fully intact. You consider peripheral nerve injury caused by intraoperative positioning of the arm. The neurology service concurs saying that this usually gets better within a day or 2.

J.G. Brock-Utne, *Case Studies of Near Misses in Clinical Anesthesia*,
DOI 10.1007/978-1-4419-1179-7_61, © Springer Science+Business Media, LLC 2011

Question

On postoperative day 5, there is unfortunately no improvement. Besides ordering a second neurology consult, is there anything else you would suggest at this stage?

Solution

Brain MRI and MRA. The Brain MRI shows an acute lacunar infarction in the posterior right frontal lobe, within the primary motor cortex serving the hand. The brain and neck MRA is unremarkable.

In this case (George V, Fielder M, Barker SJ, 2009, Postoperative arm weakness: brachial plexus injury or something else? personal communication), the patient was started on aspirin 81 mg daily. Transthoracic echocardiogram and carotid duplex studies were normal. On discharge on day 7, there was very little improvement in motor weakness of the right arm.

Perioperative stroke (POS) occurs very seldom. The incidence depends on the length of the surgical procedure, the urgency, and the amount of blood loss [1]. In cardiac surgery permanent neurological deficits due to POS may occur in 6% of patients [1, 2]. If one excludes cardiac, carotid, neck, and intracranial surgeries, the incidence of POS is 0.04–0.2% [3]. Risk factors for getting POS include previous strokes, diabetes, hypertension, peripheral vascular disease, and postoperative cardiac arrhythmias [1, 2, 4]. The predominant mechanism is embolic, with one study showing that 62% of POS patients suffered an embolic infarct after coronary artery bypass grafting. Surprisingly thrombotic, hemorrhagic, and lacunar infarcts accounted for less than 5% [1].

Recommendation

Remember that POS, although rare in patients with few risk factors, can still occur.

References

1. Selim M. Perioperative stroke. N Engl J Med. 2007;356:706–13.
2. Bucerius J et al. Stroke after cardiac surgery. A risk factor analysis of 16,184 consecutive adult patients. Ann Thorac Surg. 2003;75:472–8.
3. Brown D et al. Perioperative stroke caused by arterial tumor embolism. Anesth Analg. 2004;98:806–9.
4. Ide M et al. Early postoperative stroke in patients with an arterial septal aneurysm. Anesth Analg. 1999;89:300–1.

Chapter 62
Case 62: Persistent Intraoperative Hiccups – What to Do?

Today you are to anesthetize a 3-year-old boy, weighing 16 kg, ASA 2, with a history of congenital, bilateral profound hearing loss. He is scheduled for a cochlear implant. In the preoperative area, he is seen to be hiccupping at a constant rate of 4/min. The whole head moves vigorously. The mother informs you that the child always gets hiccups when he is nervous. You give him midazolam 8 mg per os 20 min prior to induction. You note that this has minimal effect on the hiccupping. However, he is more sedated. After application of standard monitoring, a routine inhalational induction with sevoflurane in oxygen is done. Thereafter, you establish a peripheral venous access and administration of 100 mg propofol and 50 mcg of fentanyl. The trachea is intubated with a cuffed 4.5-mm endotracheal tube. The lungs are mechanically ventilated in a pressure-controlled mode. Anesthesia is maintained with sevoflurane in air and continuous infusion of remifentanil at an infusion rate between 0.05 and 0.2 mcg/kg/min.

Unfortunately, the hiccups do not decrease during either induction or after endotracheal intubation. With maintenance of anesthesia, the hiccups actually increased to a rate of 5–7/min. You apply several circles of continuous positive airway pressure between 25 and 30 mmHg for a 10-s interval without effect [1]. A carefully placed orogastric tube [2] yields only minimal air and stomach content. This has no effect on reducing the hiccups. The manual manipulation of the vagal nerve and later the administration of 0.1 mg atropine, followed by 20 mg lidocaine, additional propofol (50 mg) and fentanyl (50 mcg) bolus, and mild hypercarbia all remains ineffective.

J.G. Brock-Utne, *Case Studies of Near Misses in Clinical Anesthesia*,
DOI 10.1007/978-1-4419-1179-7_62,

The surgeons state that they can't do the microscopic cochlea implant, due to the rigorous contractions and consecutive movement of the head. You suggest muscle paralysis but they tell you that muscular paralysis is contraindicated because of the necessity of continuous monitoring of the facial nerve. The surgeon is now considering canceling the case.

Question

Is there anything else you can suggest?

Solution

You ask the surgeon if it would be possible for him to dissect out the facial nerve despite the hiccups. If he can do that, then muscle relaxation can be given for the cochlea implant. The surgeon agreed to this plan. After the muscle relaxation was given, the hiccups stopped immediately. The operation concluded successfully. After 90 min in the postanesthesia care unit, the patient was discharged home, but still hiccupping at a rate of 5–7/min. A call to the patient's parents that evening informed us that the hiccups were terminated shortly after arriving home [3].

Perioperative hiccups have not been associated with documented increased morbidity among pediatric patients [4]. However, refractory hiccupping can interfere with surgical or diagnostic procedures, especially in cases when muscular paralysis is contraindicated as was in this case [3]. It is important to be aware that persistent intraoperative hiccupping may be the presenting feature of negative pressure pulmonary edema [4] or acid aspiration [5]. It is possible that the preoperative administration of midazolam could have increased the hiccups [6].

Recommendation

In cases where persistent intraoperative hiccups treatments fail, remember the surgeon may be able to help by allowing muscle paralysis during certain phases of the surgery.

References

1. Saitto C, Gristina G, Cosmi EV. Treatment of hiccups by continuous positive airway pressure (CPAP) in anesthetized subjects. Anesthesiology. 1982;57:345.
2. Howard SR. Persistent hiccups. BMJ. 1992;305:1237–8.
3. Panousis P, Kaufenberg Z, Brock-Utne JG. Persistent intraoperative hiccups. Remember the surgeon can help (Submitted for publications 2010).
4. Stuth EAE, Stucke AG, Berens RJ. Negative-pressure pulmonary edema in a child with hiccups during induction. Anesthesiology. 2000;93:282–4.
5. Borromeo CJ, Canes D, Stix MS, Glick ME. Hiccupping and regurgitation via the drain tube of the ProSeal Laryngeal Mask. Anesth Analg. 2002;94:1040–5.
6. Lierz P, Marhofer P, Glaser C, Krenn CG, Grabner CM, Semsroth M. Incidence and therapy of midazolam induced hiccups in pediatric anesthesia. Paediatr Anaesth. 1999;9:295–8.

Chapter 63
Case 63: Internal Jugular Cannulation

A morbidly obese male (160 kg, 5 ft 9 in.) is scheduled for a laparoscopic gastric bypass procedure. His past history is significant for high blood pressure, increased lipidemia, and difficult IV access. In the preoperative holding area, you establish a 20-G IV in the back of the wrist. You give him an antacid and take him to the operating room. A rapid sequence with metoclopramide, fentanyl, propofol, and succinylcholine is uneventful. The airway is secured with an endotracheal tube. The 20-G IV is not working well at this point. You decide to place a right internal jugular vein (IJV) catheter and call for the ultrasound machine. Unfortunately, the only two machines in the OR have been sent for repairs. The patient's neck circumference is 45 cm and this may make the insertion more difficult [1].

Question

Is there any maneuver that you can do to make the cannulation of the IJV easier?

DOI 10.1007/978-1-4419-1179-7_63,

Solution

The application of 10-cm H_2O PEEP has been shown to increase the cross-sectional area of the IJV by 41% (Hollenbeck KJ, et al., 2009, personal communication). The interesting point of this study was that the increase in the cross-sectional area of the IJV was not associated with a difference in age, gender, body mass index, NPO status, or peak inspiratory pressure. Among the several disadvantage of applying PEEP in ventilated anesthetized patients is that you may reverse the flow in a probe patent foramen ovale [2].

In a study by Fujiki et al. [1], they found that there was no statistically significant difference in the success rate of IJV puncture between morbidly obese patients and nonobese patients. Keeping the head in a neutral position, in morbidly obese patients, minimizes the overlapping of the IJV over the carotid artery.

Recommendation

Remember that PEEP may increase the cross-sectional area of the IJV.

References

1. Fujiki M, Guta C, Lemmens HJM, Brock-Utne JG. Is it more difficult to cannulate the right internal jugular vein in morbidly obese patients than in non-obese patients? Obes Surg. 2008;18:1157–9.
2. Jaffe RA, Pito FJ, Schnittgere I, Siegel LC, Wranne B, Brock-Utne JG. Aspects of mechanical ventilation affecting interatrial shunt flows during general anesthesia. Anesth Analg. 1992;75:484–8.

Chapter 64
Case 64: Endobronchial Foreign Body

You are on a medical mission to a small African country. You have just arrived. In the emergency room, you watch a stream of patients coming to be seen. The doctor on call happens to be an elderly gentleman, who does everything himself. The main reason that he does everything is that he is the only doctor in the hospital. A 16-month-old boy is admitted with increasing wheezing and stridor over the past 4 h. The child has had a history of asthma for 3–4 months, which has not got better with medical treatment. The mother accompanying the child says this is the worst he has been. Chest exam exhibits the classical asthma signs. He is frightened and distressed. You hear him wheezing with each forced exhalation. He does not look cyanosed. There is no pulse oximeter in the emergency room. He is using accessory muscles and there is decreased air entry to the right lung. The chest X-ray shows some evidence of atelectasis in the lower right lobe. Your new friend, the doctor in the emergency department, diagnoses a possible foreign body aspiration. He books the child for a bronchoscopy in the main operating room. He is going to do the case with a nonanesthesia-trained assistant. You offer your services as an anesthesiologist. The doctor is delighted.

In the operating room, you perform an uneventful inhalation induction. Peripheral IV access is started with a 22-G IV in the hand. A ridged bronchoscopy identifies a foreign body in the right main bronchus. Multiple attempts, by the doctor, to remove it both with forceps and suction catheters prove unsuccessful. The doctor is not comfortable to do a thoracotomy.

Question

With the child still anesthetized, what would you suggest as a possibility to get the foreign body out?

J.G. Brock-Utne, *Case Studies of Near Misses in Clinical Anesthesia*,
DOI 10.1007/978-1-4419-1179-7_64, © Springer Science+Business Media, LLC 2011

Solution

You placed a 2.0 Fogarty catheter through the bronchoscope in the deflated position [1]. The catheter was slipped past the foreign body and the balloon inflated. By pulling on the Fogarty catheter, a solid metal object was dislodged and removed with a forceps. A flexible bronchoscope was introduced and no other foreign bodies were seen. The patient was awakened and had an uneventful recovery and was discharged home the next day.

One should be aware that complications have been reported with the use of the Fogarty catheter in this manner [2, 3]. These include balloon rupture and/or catheter tip rupture. If that occurs then most likely an invasive approach must be done. These complications are thankfully rare.

It is important to realize that if the history indicates that the foreign body could for example be a peanut, then this is a real emergency. Peanuts being an organic matter and very salty will absorb water and swell causing sudden airway obstruction with disastrous results. This is especially true if the peanut is in the trachea. I have personally seen this and we were very lucky to have a live child at the end of the procedure.

Recommendation

The Fogarty catheter has several functions and this is one of them.

References

1. Mackle T, Russell J. The combined use of Fogarty balloon with extraction forceps for the controlled retrieval of an endobronchial foreign body. Int J Pediatr Otorhinolaryngol. 2001;60:163–5.
2. Treen DC, Falterman KW, Arensman RM. Complications of the Fogarty catheter technique for removal of endobronchial foreign bodies. J Pediatr Surg. 1989;24:613–5.
3. Ross MN, Haase GM. An alternative approach to management of Fogarty catheter disruption associated with endobronchial foreign body extraction. Chest. 1988;94:882–4.

Chapter 65
Case 65: A Cyst in Fourth Ventricle

A 15-year-old boy (60 kg, 5 ft) presents for the removal of a neurocysticercosis cyst from the fourth ventricle. The surgical approach is a transsphenoidal approach. The patient is otherwise healthy, with no allergies. General anesthesia is induced in a routine manner. Anesthesia maintenance is with N_2O in oxygen with isoflurane 0.6% and remifentanil 0.05 μg/kg/min. The surgery is progressing as planned. Unfortunately after opening the fourth ventricle, the surgeons find it very difficult to remove the cyst.

Question

Is there anything you can do to help the surgeon remove the cyst?

J.G. Brock-Utne, *Case Studies of Near Misses in Clinical Anesthesia*,
DOI 10.1007/978-1-4419-1179-7_65, © Springer Science+Business Media, LLC 2011

Solution

Valsalva's maneuver (VM). Studies have shown that VM can increase intracranial pressure in neurosurgical patients [1, 2]. In a case report (3), VM resulted in extrusion of an intracranial cyst. This made it possible for the surgeon to pass an irrigation catheter behind the cyst. When saline was injected through the catheter, the adhesions behind the cyst reduced to such an extent that the cyst was removed intact. The rest of the surgery was uneventful.

Recommendation

Valsalva maneuver is often used in patients undergoing intracranial surgery to confirm venous hemostats. It can also be used to facilitate tumor/cyst removal during transsphenoidal pituitary surgery.

References

1. Prabhaker H, Bithal PK, Suri A, Rath GP, Dash HH. Intracranial pressure changes during Valsalva maneuver in patients undergoing neuroendoscopic procedures. Minim Invasive Neurosurg. 2007;50:98–101.
2. Wendling W, Sadel S, Jimenez D, Rosenwasser R, Buchheit W. Cardiovascular and cerebrovascular effects of applied Valsalva maneuver in neurosurgical patients. Eur J Anaesthesiol. 1994;11:81–7.

Chapter 66
Case 66: Generalized Convulsions After Regional Anesthesia

A 28-year-old man (78 kg, 5 ft 10 in.) is admitted to hospital in the early morning. He has sustained a cut in his right ulnar nerve following a knife fight with a "friend." You examine him carefully and see no other injuries especially no other knife injuries. He is under the influence of alcohol and states that he has neither eaten nor drunk anything for the last 5 h. He denies having any allergies to drugs. His vital signs are stable and his hemoglobin is 11 g%. He has no fixed address and denies any medical problems or illicit drug use. He arrives in the operating room with an IV infusion of lactated Ringer's solution. He has received a total of 1 L since admission 1 h earlier. You place at 4:00 a.m. a supraclavicular brachial plexus block with a mixture of 1.5 mg/kg (20 mL) bupivacaine 0.5% and 1.5 mg/kg lidocaine 1% (10 mL). At 4:20 a.m., surgery starts. The patient feels no pain. Five minutes later, 4:25 a.m., the patient develops what appear to be general convulsions. However, he is breathing, and oxygen saturation remains within acceptable limits above 95 with 100% via an oxygen mask. His heart rate is 94 regular and his BP is 140/90.

The surgeon has now stopped working, since the patient, but not the injured arm, is moving.

Question

What is the possible diagnosis and what will you do?

J.G. Brock-Utne, *Case Studies of Near Misses in Clinical Anesthesia*,
DOI 10.1007/978-1-4419-1179-7_66, © Springer Science+Business Media, LLC 2011

Solutions

Differential diagnosis

1. Toxic reaction to the local anesthetic drugs. Unlikely. The length of time from the injection of the drugs to the onset of convulsions is too long even for a delayed onset caused by slow absorption (25 min).
2. Undiagnosed epileptic. Unlikely. He did not show the classic signs such a tongue biting and/or incontinence.
3. Hypoglycemic coma caused by excessive and prolonged alcohol intake. Likely.

In this case, you inject 50% dextrose solution with good effect. The patient stops convulsing and becomes rational and the surgery is concluded under the supraclavicular block.

In a previous case [1], a 22-year-old man with a history of excessive alcohol intake developed delayed convulsions after a regional block. In that case, the convulsions subsided over a 10-min period after the administrations of IV glucose. The patient's blood glucose level after receiving 60 mL of 50% dextrose was 2.3 mmol/L (normal fasting levels, 3.33–6.60 mmol/L).

If this diagnosis had been missed, the patient could have been treated in two ways, both dangerous to him.

1. Given a general anesthetic, since he would not lie still.
2. Wrongly treated for a toxic reaction to local anesthetics (e.g., paralyzing and ventilating the patient).

In both cases, serious brain damage would have occurred if IV glucose was not given.

Recommendation

Excessive alcohol intake can cause hypoglycemia. If this diagnosis is missed, serious brain damage may result.

Reference

1. Naidu R, Brock-Utne JG. Generalized convulsion following regional anesthesia – a pertinent lesson. Anesth Analg. 1988;67:1192.

Chapter 67
Case 67: Cardiac Arrest in a Prone Patient

A 28-year-old male (84 kg, 5 ft 11 in.) is admitted to hospital with pelvic fractures. He was run over by a train. His past history is significant for depression. Otherwise he is healthy and has no allergies. On examination he is awake, but in severe pain. No other injuries are found. Examination of this heart and lung reveals nothing abnormal. His chest X-ray is normal. He is taken to the operating room for an open reduction internal fixation (ORIF) for his multiple pelvic fractures in a prone position. A rapid sequence induction is performed uneventfully with etomidate and succinylcholine. The airway is secured with #8 endotracheal tube. Maintenance of anesthesia is with N_2O in oxygen, sevoflurane, and fentanyl. Before the patient is turned prone, a right radial artery line, an internal jugular vein (Arrow-Flex sheath 9Fr, Arrow International, Reading, PA 19605), and a 14-G peripheral line are inserted. The operation proceeds uneventfully and the blood loss of 5 L has been replaced. The arterial blood gases and electrolytes are normal, with an HCT of 28%. Heart rate is 80 bpm, BP 110/75, and the central venous pressure (CVP) is 15 cm H_2O. Within a minute of having recorded these parameters, there is sudden loss in arterial blood pressure tracing, a rapid decrease in end-tidal CO_2 and oxygen saturation. The EKG showed a sinus rhythm of 130 bpm, but there are no carotid pulses.

Questions

What will you do?

1. Turn the patient quickly supine and institute CPR?
2. Attempt to do CPR in the prone position and then turn the patient supine?

J.G. Brock-Utne, *Case Studies of Near Misses in Clinical Anesthesia*,
DOI 10.1007/978-1-4419-1179-7_67,

Solution

Attempt CPR in the prone position. Several case reports have suggested that prone position should be considered as the optimal choice for CPR in certain limited circumstances, even if the supine position is achievable [1]. I believe that prone CPR must be started immediately. This will hopefully provide oxygenation to the brain and heart while everyone gets ready to turn the patient supine.

In the case above (Almazan D and Tzabazis A, 2009, personal communication), prone CPR was started immediately. The surgeon placed both palms below the lower border of the patient's scapula and performed chest compression. Since the patient was on a frame that supported his anterior thorax, there was no need for counter pressures. Systolic pressures of over 80 mmHg (seen from the arterial wave form) were easily achieved. Within 2 min, 1 mg of epinephrine and 0.4 mg of atropine were given IV. Spontaneous return of cardio pulmonary function occurred as the patient was turned supine. He was taken to the ICU. Thirty minutes later, he was following commands. Further medical workup identified the cause of the pulseless electrical activity (PEA) arrest as a pulmonary embolus. The surgical operation was completed 3 days later after an IVC filter had been placed. He was subsequently discharged from the hospital with his prior preoperative neurological status intact. In this case, the effective prone CPR saved his life as vaso-active medications were allowed to circulate with visual improvement to oxygen saturation, arterial blood pressure, and end-tidal CO_2.

In cases where there is no counter-pressure available, a clenched left fist must be placed under the sternum while the right hand compresses the mid-thoracic spine. Ideally, the prone CPR should be done by two persons, one doing the counter-pressure and the other doing the compression.

Risk factors for intraoperative cardiac arrest in patients in the prone position include the following: cardiac abnormalities, hypovolemia, air embolism, wound irrigation with hydrogen peroxide, poor positioning, and occluded venous return [2].

Mazer et al. [3], in a pilot study, concluded that prone CPR generated sufficient mean blood pressures.

Recommendation

Fortunately, cardiac arrest in the prone anesthetized patient is rare. However, when it occurs you must attempt the best prone CPR that you and the surgeon can muster before the patient is turned supine. If you have an arterial line, you can monitor the CPR effectiveness.

References

1. Beltran SL, Mashour GA. Unsuccessful cardiopulmonary resuscitation during neurosurgery: is the supine position always optimal? Anesthesiology. 2008;108:163–4.
2. Brown J, Rogers J, Soar J. Cardiac arrest during surgery and ventilation in the prone position: a case report and systematic review. Resuscitation. 2001;50:233–8.
3. Mazer SP, Weisfeldt M, Bai D, Carinale C, Arora R, Ma C, et al. Reverse CPR: a pilot study of CPR in the prone position. Resuscitation. 2003;57:279–85.

Chapter 68
Case 68: A Short Patient with a High BMI

Today you are scheduled to anesthetize a very pleasant 44-year-old lady. She is 145 kg and 4 ft 9 in. (BMI 56.3). She is coming for a vaginal hysterectomy. She is otherwise healthy with no allergies. You place an IV in the preoperative area, give her sedation, and take her to the operating room. You anesthetize her in a routine fashion. She is an easy mask and a grade 2 view. The airway is secured with a #7 endotracheal tube and bilateral air entry is heard. After the patient is asleep, the patient's legs are positioned in stirrups (Yellowfins, Allen Medical, Acton, MA 01720). Prior to the start of the operation, the surgeon requests the operating room table to be elevated as high possible, with a steep head down position. She explains that this is done so that she, the surgeon, can stand and see what she is doing.

The operating table is elevated to the level of your face; thereafter, the patient is placed in a steep Trendelenburg position. You sit down on your chair; your knees are now just below the patient's head.

Questions

Would you be concerned? If so why?

J.G. Brock-Utne, *Case Studies of Near Misses in Clinical Anesthesia*,
DOI 10.1007/978-1-4419-1179-7_68, © Springer Science+Business Media, LLC 2011

Solution

At the time I was not concerned. I was sitting at the head of the table beside the anesthesia machine. Approximately 40 min into the case, with the surgeons looking at their instruments and not the operating site, the patient start to slide down the table. I tried to hold her but could not. She just kept sliding. Before I knew what had happened, I was sitting on the floor with the patient's head in my lap and the right hand holding the ETT. To my relief, her vital signs remained unchanged. Since the surgeon was not looking and this all happened very quietly, the first thing I heard was the surgeon saying: "Where did the patient go?" I did not know what to say but I think I said: "She is down here, can someone get me another anesthesiologist?" My friend and colleague Dr. Alex Macario appeared and looked at me and said: "What are you doing down there?"

The patient was repositioned, but this time the step Trendelenburg was not used.

No study could be found as to the fall rate of anesthetized patients from operating room tables. However, in-hospital-falls is not uncommon [1–3]. In one study in a large academic hospital found that the fall rate was 3.1 falls per 1,000 patient-days [1]. The rate varied by service. Some 6.1% of falls resulted in serious injuries [1]. Most common injuries were bleeding or laceration (53.6%), fracture or dislocation (15.9%), and hematoma or contusion (13%) [1].

Recommendation

You must watch out for patients, who have small appendages, placed in stirrups and in a steep Trendelenburg. Patients like this can slide off the operating table with potentially disastrous results.

References

1. Fisher ID, Krauss MJ, Claiborne Dunagan W, Birge S, Hitcho E, Johnson S, et al. Patterns and predictors of inpatient falls and fall-related injuries in a large academic hospital. Infect Control Hosp Epidemiol. 2005;26:822–7.
2. Inouye SK, Brown CJ, Tinetti ME. Medicare nonpayment, hospital falls, and unintended consequences. N Engl J Med. 2009;360:2390–2.
3. Von Renteln-Kruse W, Krause T. Incidence of in-hospital falls in geriatric patients before and after the introduction of an interdisciplinary team-based fall-prevention intervention. J Am Geriatr Soc. 2007;55:2068–74.

Chapter 69
Case 69: Bleeding After Oral Surgery

A 55-year-old man (74 kg, 5 ft 11 in.) is admitted with a painful ulcerative lesion in the left retromolar area. The lesion is 1.5 cm. A biopsy of the lesion under local anesthesia 2 days ago has revealed a carcinoma in situ. He is scheduled today for a wide excision with periosteal stripping of the mandible. He has a long history of depression for which he takes sertraline (a selective serotonin reuptake inhibitor (SSRI)) 100 mg daily. Since he has had a lot of pain, he has been taking naproxen (a nonsteroidal anti-inflammatory drug) 500 mg twice daily. He also smokes about 20 cigarettes and drinks 5 units of alcohol/day. He denies other medical concerns and he has no allergies. Physical exam is none contributory. His EKG and laboratory results are all normal including the coagulation results. He is very nervous and you give him 6 mg of midazolam prior to coming to the operating room. You anesthetize him in a routine manner with fentanyl, propofol, and rocuronium. His airway is secured with an oral endotracheal tube. The anesthesia maintenance is with N_2O in 30% oxygen and desflurane. At the end of surgery, the wound is closed and hemostasis is achieved. The patient's MAP at the time of closing was 10% below the starting MAP. The patient is taken to the recovery room awake, pain free, and with stable vital signs. An hour later you are called stat to the recovery room. You find the patient in severe respiratory distress. He states he cannot breathe and is pointing to his neck. The oxygen saturation is now 90%. You discover a large hematoma in the floor of the mouth obstructing his airway. His saturation falls further to 85%. You give him an oxygen face mask and a jaw thrust but to no avail. You call for a fiberoptic cart and an ENT surgeon to do a possible tracheostomy. While you wait you attempt a blind nasal intubation. Not only are you unsuccessful but you cause an epistaxis. However, the nasal tube, now placed in the posterior pharynx, improves his oxygenation. The saturation returns to 90%. The surgeon arrives before the fiberoptic cart and successful does a tracheostomy under local anesthesia.

J.G. Brock-Utne, *Case Studies of Near Misses in Clinical Anesthesia*,
DOI 10.1007/978-1-4419-1179-7_69,

Question

What can be the cause of the hematoma, if it is not surgical, remembering that his preoperative coagulation studies were normal?

Solution

The hematoma was caused by the combination of SSRI (sertraline) and the nonsteroidal anti-inflammatory drug naproxen [1]. After the tracheostomy, the hematoma did not increase due mainly to a tamponade effect. The SSRI and naproxen were stopped and codeine prescribed with good effect. In the case report [1], a more careful medical history revealed that this patient had three episodes of abnormal bleeding after surgical procedures while on sertraline. One was after a nasal septal surgery, the other after a tooth extraction, and lastly after the biopsy of the ulcerative lesion.

SSRI causes postoperative bleeding, due to the ability of drugs to block the uptake of serotonin into the thrombocytes [1]. One of the functions of serotonin in thrombocytes is to promote platelet aggregation. When serotonin levels are depleted after several weeks of treatment, the altered platelet function leads to prolonged bleeding time. The bleeding time was not tested in this patient preoperatively mainly because it is no longer considered a reliable test. SSRI has been associated with abnormal bleeding, especially with upper gastrointestinal hemorrhage [2, 3]. A meta-analysis showed that SSRIs more than double the risk of upper gastrointestinal hemorrhage [4]. It is noteworthy that the drugs with the highest degree of serotonin reuptake inhibition – fluoxetine, paroxetine, and sertraline – are more frequently associated with abnormal bleeding [5, 6]. In surgery the risk of abnormal bleeding associated with the SSRIs is not clear, since there is a paucity of data. In orthopedic surgery, there was a fourfold risk of bleeding, while in coronary artery bypass surgery there was no such finding.

Other SSRI patients potentially at risk of abnormal bleeding would be patients receiving neuraxial blockade or patients undergoing surgery in enclosed spaces like neurosurgery.

Recommendation

It would seem prudent to be aware of a possible risk of abnormal bleeding in surgical patients taking SSRI with or without nonsteroidal anti-inflammatory drugs.

References

1. Van Cann EM, Koole R. Abnormal bleeding after an oral surgical procedure leading to airway compromise in a patient taking a selective serotonin reuptake inhibitor and a nonsteroidal anti-inflammatory drug. Anesthesiology. 2008;109:568–9.
2. Turner MS, May DB, Arthus RR, Xiong GI. Clinical impact of selective serotonin reuptake inhibitors therapy with bleeding risks. J Intern Med. 2007;261:205–13.

3. Wessinger S, Kaplan M, Choi L, Williams M, Lau C, Sharp L, et al. Increased use of selective serotonin reuptake inhibitors in patients admitted with gastrointestinal haemorrhage A multi-center retrospective analysis. Aliment Pharmacol Ther. 2006;23:937–44.
4. Luke YK, Trivedi AN, Singh S. Meta-analysis: gastrointestinal bleeding due to interaction between selective serotonin uptake inhibitors and non-steroidal anti-inflammatory drugs. Aliment Pharmacol Ther. 2008;27:31–40.
5. Halperin D, Reber G. Influence of antidepressants on hemostatsis. Dialogues Clin Neurosci. 2007;9:47–59.
6. Meijer WEE, Heerdink ER, Nlen WA, Herings RMC, Leufkens HGM, Egberts ACG. Association of risks of abnormal bleeding with degree of serotonin reuptake inhibition by antidepressants. Arch Intern Med. 2004;164:2367–70.

Chapter 70
Case 70: Selecting the Right Size Double Lumen Tube

Today you are scheduled to anesthetize a 36-year-old lady (70 kg, 5 ft 4 in.) for right upper lobectomy for chronic atelectasis. Eighteen months before she had undergone successfully a heart and bilateral lung transplant. She has no other comorbidities.

The patient's tracheal width measured 19 cm on the preoperative chest X-ray. The left bronchus was not seen on the chest X-ray. The chest computed tomography scan confirmed the tracheal width to be 19 mm and the left bronchus to be 10 mm. A tracheal width of more than 18 mm mandates a #41Fr double lumen tube (DLT) [1].

Question

Would a #41Fr be a good choice in this patient?

DOI 10.1007/978-1-4419-1179-7_70,

Solution

No. A smaller tube is required in this case.

The technique for selection of the left DLT is based on the work by Brodsky et al. [1]. However, selecting a left DLT for a patient with a lung transplant is an exception to this rule [2]. In the latter case [2], the author placed a #39Fr left DLT instead of #41Fr. The #39Fr functioned perfectly for the operation which was concluded successfully.

Normally, a trachea measuring 19 mm, with a predicted left bronchial width of >12 mm, would need a #41Fr left DLT. However, this patient's lung had been transplanted to the last distal ring of her native trachea. Also the transplanted left bronchus was smaller (10 mm) than predicted. Therefore, a 39Fr left DLT was selected. For normal patients with tracheas ≥16 mm, a 39Fr DLT is used; for tracheal diameters ≥15 mm, a 37Fr DLT is used; and for tracheal diameter <15 mm, a 35Fr DLT is used.

The recommended correct size DLT (see above) is advised [1, 2] since they can't be advanced so deeply into the airway, have less resistance to airflow during one lung ventilation, and require less air to inflate the bronchial cuff.

Recommendation

Patients who have undergone a lung transplant will most likely require a smaller than recommended left DLT.

References

1. Brodsky JB, Macario A, Mark JBD. Tracheal diameter predicts double-lumen tube size: a method for selecting left double-lumen tubes. Anesth Analg. 1996;82:861–4.
2. Habibi A, Mackey S, Brodsky JB. Selecting a double-lumen tube after lung transplant. Anesth Analg. 1997;84:938–43.

Chapter 71
Case 71: A Low Normal Preoperative Blood Glucose Level

A 48-year-old obese female (160 kg, 5 ft 4 in.) presents for a laparoscopic gastric bypass procedure. She is the first patient on the list. You see her at 7 a.m. She is a noninsulin-dependent diabetic for which she takes oral antidiabetic medication. She has hypertension and hyperlipidemia. Both are well controlled on medication. She states that her exercise tolerance is limited due to her weight. The EKG shows normal sinus rhythm. On further questioning she also takes ginseng (a herbal medicine) to "calm her nerves." This morning (5 a.m.) she has taken her antihypertensive medication and a triple dose of ginseng as she is very "nervous." On examination her chest is clear and the heart rate is 88 bpm and the BP is 140/90. You review the laboratory results and note that the electrolytes, PTT, PT, INR, and HCT are all normal. A finger stick glucose taken at 7 a.m. is 65 mg% (70–100 mg/dL). She claims that her glucose normally runs low. She confirms that has not taken her antidiabetic medication. The operation is scheduled for 4 h.

Questions

1. Are you concerned about the low blood glucose results? If so, what are you going to do about it?
2. Could there be a reason for this low normal level?

J.G. Brock-Utne, *Case Studies of Near Misses in Clinical Anesthesia*,
DOI 10.1007/978-1-4419-1179-7_71,

Solutions

One should always be concerned about low glucose levels. The triple dose of ginseng caused the hypoglycemia. This is a herbal medicine from the roots of plants from the Araliaceae family. The active constituents are ginsenosides. Ginseng has been reported as both decreasing and increasing blood pressure; acts as a central nervous system stimulant and interfere with platelet aggregation. Asian ginseng is obtained from Panax ginseng. The name Panax is derived from the Greek panacea, meaning cure-all.

Lanca [1] has reported several adverse effects and drug interactions caused by ginseng. These include the following:

1. Both in vitro and in vivo studies have shown ginseng to reduce blood glucose levels. Ginseng action is to stimulate the insulin synthesis and regulate intestinal absorption of glucose. Hence ginseng should be used cautiously in patients with type 2 diabetes who are also taking oral hypoglycemic drugs.
2. Anticoagulant properties of ginseng have also been reported. Of interest is the fact that ginseng in a randomized controlled clinical trial increased the risk of blood clotting in patients treated with warfarin.
3. Interactions with MAO inhibitors.

Recommendation

There is an increased use of herbal medicine. Knowledge of herbal medication and especially of the adverse effects and drug interactions is imperative when anesthetizing patients who take herbal medications.

Reference

1. Lanca J. Herbal medications: an evidence-based review. CME Calif Physicians. 2008;134: 19–42.

Chapter 72
Case 72: Things to Remember When You Change a Cordis Catheter to a Triple Lumen

You are called late at night to change a Cordis Catheter (Arrow Flex Sheath, 9Fr), situated in a patient's internal jugular vein (IJV) to a triple lumen. Both catheters are made by Arrow, Reading, PA 19605. This is not your patient but you are the first call and everyone has gone home. The patient is awake in the recovery room. Her past history is significant for obesity, hypertension, insulin-dependent diabetes mellitus, coronary artery disease with angioplasty and bypass grafting, and deep vein thrombosis. She was originally going to ICU but is now being admitted to an ordinary ward. Since the hospital policy is that no patient can have a cordis in an ordinary ward, the cordis must either be removed or changed to a triple lumen. The surgeon wants a triple lumen for IV access, as she has no other IV working.

In these cases you must always be sure that:

1. The change-over is done with the patient in the head down position.
2. The cordis wound looks clear and there is no hematoma.
3. The clothing profile is normal.
4. You have another working IV.
5. The procedure is done with a sterile technique.
6. You know that the Cordis has an 8Fr obturator, which is attached to a twist-lock.
7. You understand that the spring wire guide used for the catheter exchange will puncture the diaphragm on the proximal end of the Arrow Flex Sheath. This could lead to excessive bleeding.
8. You ask the patient to take a deep breath when you remove the cordis.

Question

You are about to proceed but there seems to be something important that you have forgotten. What could that be?

J.G. Brock-Utne, *Case Studies of Near Misses in Clinical Anesthesia*,
DOI 10.1007/978-1-4419-1179-7_72, © Springer Science+Business Media, LLC 2011

Solution

Make sure there is no prior placement of an inferior vena cava (IVC) jugular filter [1]. This can be done by asking the patient, look at the record or the chest X-ray. This is especially true of a patient who has a history of deep vein thrombosis. In the case report [1], the triple lumen guide wire was advanced approximately 50 cm into the IJV. The triple lumen catheter was advanced over the guide wire without any problems. However, the guide wire got entangled with the filter making it nearly impossible to remove it. Eventually, it was removed forcefully. After the guide wire was removed, a chest X-ray showed the IVC filter in the superior vena cava. Luckily, the displaced filter was removed through a filter sheath without complications.

To avoid this type of complication in a patient with an IVC filter, it is essential that the guide wire is inserted only 10 cm into the IJV.

Remember that the IVC filter can easily be seen on a chest X-ray. A chest X-ray taken earlier in this case [1] showed the filter in the correct position.

On another note, it is obviously important to remove the guide wire after placing any central venous catheter. This is recorded in a case report from China [2]. The guide wire, which was accidentally lost during insertion of a subclavian vein catheter insertion, was discovered protruding from the patient's back of neck 6 months after the event. The author reports that the catheter was easily removed from his neck.

Recommendation

It is a good idea to only insert the guide wire no more than 10 cm into the IJV.

References

1. Sudip N, Stockoz-Scaff L. A complication of central venous catheterization. N Engl J Med. 2007;356:21.
2. Guo H. Complication of central venous catheterization. N Engl J Med. 2007;356:1075.

Chapter 73
Case 73: An Intraoperative Malfunctioning Vaporizer

It is Monday morning and you are scheduled to give anesthesia in a surgical clinic. Your list consists of four gynecological cases. The first patient is a 30-year-old woman (78 kg, 5 ft 8 in.) with a diagnosis of pelvic pain. She is admitted for a removal of an adnexal mass. The patient is otherwise healthy with no past surgical history. She takes only "over the counter analgesics" for her pain. You see her in the preoperative holding area. After an IV is placed and 3 mg of midazolam IV is given, she is taken to the operating room. After preoxygenation, the patient is anesthetized with propofol, fentanyl, and vecuronium. For maintenance you select sevoflurane in air (50%) and oxygen. You give the nurse permission to catheterize the patient. The vital signs are stable but you notice that the end expired sevoflurane value is only 0.5% even though the patient has now been on sevoflurane 2% for at least 5 min. You check that the vaporizer is full and that it is sitting correctly. You increase the sevoflurane to 6% but the end-tidal sevoflurane value stays at 0.5% even after 10 min. You are now concerned that the patient may become aware, so you review the vital signs. The heart rate has increased from 78 to 88 bpm and the BP has increased from 110/80 to 145/90. The pupils are 2.5 mm (not pinpoint). The surgeon has just made his incision and is happily working away.

Question

What will you do?

J.G. Brock-Utne, *Case Studies of Near Misses in Clinical Anesthesia*,
DOI 10.1007/978-1-4419-1179-7_73, © Springer Science+Business Media, LLC 2011

Solution

You must prevent, at all cost, the patient having an intraoperative awareness. In this case I would:

1. Change from sevoflurane to another inhalational agent. In this case isoflurane.
2. Add nitrous oxide – 70% in oxygen.
3. Disconnect the endotracheal tube from the Y and see if you can smell sevoflurane. This is to inform the anesthetic technician (if there is one in the surgery center) that either the capnograph or the vaporizer is wrong. It is unlikely that both have failed at the same time. If you hardly smell any vapor then the vaporizer must be replaced.
4. Give more analgesics.
5. See if the end-tidal isoflurane concentration rises to reasonable values.
6. If it does check with your nose that you have isoflurane.
7. Keep a close eye on the patient's vital signs. They should normalize. Check also the pupils. They should get smaller if you are successful in adequately anesthetizing the patient.
8. If you are not happy that the patient is adequately asleep, tell the surgeon to stop, so you can get ready to employ a total intravenous anesthetic technique.
9. If you are concerned that the patient may be aware, then you must talk to the patient, tell them that they may be aware, but everything is fine etc. I had a case where I thought the patient (690 lb man) was aware due to a large sudden blood loss necessitating turning the inhalational agent down. The patient could after the surgery, a few hours later, tell me exactly what I had said. Since he had a working thoracic epidural, he had no pain but he claimed he was comforted by my voice. The episode lasted no more than 5–10 min. Six months later, at X-mas, he sent me a hand-knitted scarf.
10. At the end of the anesthetic, wheel the whole anesthesia machine out into the corridor and ask for a new one. It is unlikely that there is a fulltime anesthetic technician in a "free standing" surgical clinic. If there is, it is further unlikely that he/she can fix the machine/vaporizer. Hence you do not want to take any chances.
11. Postoperatively, you establish if the patient was aware. If so you should get the Risk/Management team involved. Remember to explain (in the presence of witnesses) what happened not only to the patient but also to any family member. Make good notes.
12. Find out what was the matter with the machine/vaporizer.

This happened to a friend of mine. He changed to isoflurane after about 10 min. Unfortunately, the patient could recall the insertion of the urinary catheter. The patient was informed about the machine failure and was satisfied with the explanation and did not press charges.

I strongly believe in the size of the pupil as an indication that the patient is anesthetized. A small to pinpoint pupil is most likely a sign that the patient is asleep.

Do be aware that drugs like phenylephrine in large doses IV can cause mydriasis (dilation of the pupil). The mydriasis is caused by the sympathetic nervous system fibers to the eye exciting the radial fibers of the iris leading to dilation of the pupil.

Recommendation

You must physically remove the whole anesthesia machine from the operating room and refuse to use it anymore until it is checked out. Make a note of the anesthesia machine serial number. This incident must be report IN WRITING to the director of the operating room. Send a copy to your anesthesia group and keep a copy for yourself. By not filing a written report, the machine could be used the next day. If the machine is used and a disaster occurs, you may be accused of not having reported the problem.

Chapter 74
Case 74: An Abnormal EKG First Discovered in the Operating Room

A 59 year old accountant (69 kg, 5 ft 8 in.) is admitted as an outpatient for a cholecystectomy. Five days previously he was admitted with gallstone pancreatitis. An ERCP with sphincterotomy was done 3 days ago under general anesthesia with no complications. The patient was discharged home the same day. His past medical history is significant for hypertension which is well controlled. He exercises as a coach for a Christian Youth Soccer league. His mother is still alive at 92 but his father died of heart disease at 72. You meet the patient in the preoperative holding area and place an IV. His only EKG in the chart was taken on admission 5 days ago. It shows minimal ST depression in lateral leads with a regular sinus rhythm of 79 bpm. His BP is 130/85 mmHg. He is a bit anxious and you sedate him with midazolam 3 mg IV and take him to the operating room. After positioning the patient on the operating room table, noninvasive monitoring is placed. You look in amazement at the EKG strip generated by your Datex Monitor – shown in Fig. 74.1.

His vital signs are heart rate 76 bpm and BP 113/73. You turn to the patient who is seen to be relaxing with closed eyes and you ask him: "Have you any chest pain or difficulty in breathing at the moment?" To which he declares: "No, I feel very relaxed and comfortable."

The surgeon now walks in and wonders why the patient is not asleep.

J.G. Brock-Utne, *Case Studies of Near Misses in Clinical Anesthesia*,
DOI 10.1007/978-1-4419-1179-7_74, © Springer Science+Business Media, LLC 2011

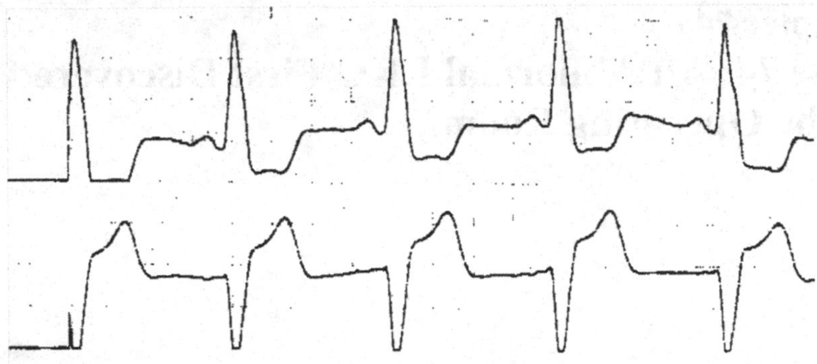

Fig. 74.1 EKG strip

Question

What will you do?

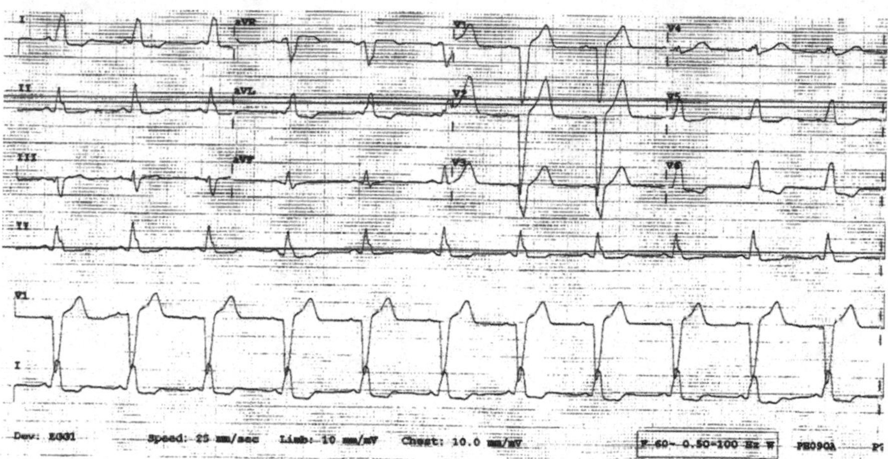

Fig. 74.2 EKG trace

Solution

This case happened to me.

I explained to the surgeon that the patient had developed a new onset of left bundle branch block (LBBB). As we stood looking at the EKG trace it reverts back to its normal configuration as seen on his EKG from 5 days ago. The heart rate was 68 bpm and BP 102/71. Three to five minutes later the EKG was as shown in Fig. 74.2 with evidence of LBBB.

The case was canceled and the patient taken to the recovery room. Here, a 12 lead EKG reveals sinus rhythm with LBBB. Cardiology was called to evaluate. They performed a carotid massage which broke the LBBB. Thus, a rate dependent LBBB was diagnosed. He was discharged home and referred for further cardiac workup.

So the question was: When did LBBB first occur? It could have been intermittent for a long time or maybe only since the ERCP? Had a 12 lead EKG been done prior to this operation, an LBBB could have been diagnosed. If so, he would not have been taken to the operating room. A cardiac consult would have been sought immediately.

Recommendation

A new onset LBBB must always be taken seriously. Further cardiac workup is essential.

Chapter 75
Case 75: A Cardiac Arrest in ICU

You are called urgently in the middle of the night to the ICU to assist with cardiopulmonary resuscitation. A medical student, who knows the patient, runs to you. He tells you that the patient is a 41-year-old man with a history of dilated cardiomyopathy. He has undergone a heart transplant 5 days ago. On postoperative day 2, he developed multiorgan dysfunction requiring multiple vasopressors and ionotropic agents to maintain hemodynamic stability. He has been sedated continuously with propofol and has a working radial line catheter.

When you arrive, a nurse is doing heart compression and the respiratory therapist is hand ventilating the patient's lungs with 100% oxygen. The patient has developed a pulseless ventricular tachycardic arrest. His only IV access is a triple lumen (Arrow, Reading, PA 19605) inserted into the right subclavian vein. Each line, as it emerges from the patient, has a stopcock attached to it. You disconnect the propofol infusion that is attached to a stopcock on the most distal line of the triple lumen. Resuscitation drugs are injected 30 cm more distal through this stopcock. No effect is seen. You easily aspirate blood from the distal lumen, but note that the patient's hospital gown over his right shoulder is wet. All the stopcocks close to the triple lumen are inserted tightly but the stopcock that has been used to infuse propofol is damp. You replace this stopcock and the patient is successfully resuscitated.

Question

Can you think of a reason why the stopcock failed?

J.G. Brock-Utne, *Case Studies of Near Misses in Clinical Anesthesia*,
DOI 10.1007/978-1-4419-1179-7_75,

Solution

The stopcock that had been used to infuse propofol was later found to have a crack in it (Matthew Kolz and John L Chow, personal communication 2004). Studies have shown that lipid-based infusions and propofol can cause cracks in stopcocks [1, 2]. However, ICUs should have stopcocks that can be used safely with the above solutions. It is possible that the cracked stopcock mentioned above came from the operating room and was not changed when the patient arrived in the ICU.

Since propofol has become popular in ICU sedation [2–4], the clinician must be aware of this problem.

Recommendation

Only use stopcocks that do not crack when lipid-based medications including propofol are employed.

References

1. Nakao M, Yamanaka S, Onji I. Cracks of polycarbonate three-way stopcock are caused by fat emulsion not by propofol. Masui. 2000;49:802–5 (Article in Japanese).
2. Nakao M, Yamanaka S, Iwata M, Nakashima M, Onji I. The cracks of polycarbonate three-way stopcocks are enhanced by the lubricating action of fat emulsion of propofol. Masui. 2003;52:1243–7 (Article in Japanese).
3. Hall RI, Sandham D, Carinal P, Tweeddale M, Moher D, Wang X, et al. Propofol vs midazolam for ICU sedation: a Canadian multicenter randomized trial. Chest. 2001;119:1151–9.
4. Young C, Knudsen N, Hilton A, Reves JG. Sedation in the intensive care unit. Crit Care Med. 2000;28:854–66.

Chapter 76
Case 76: A Severe Case of Metabolic Acidosis

A 48-year-old otherwise healthy female (68 kg and 5 ft 7 in.) with Moyamoya disease is scheduled for an extracranial–intracranial revascularization (EC–IC bypass). She has a past history of hypertension and hyperlipidemia. Her kidney function is deemed normal. She is having this procedure since she has had transient ischemic episodes recently. Five days prior to the surgery, she stopped taking Clopidogrel (Plavix). She is admitted the day before surgery for a Single-Photon Emission CT scan (SPECT scan). Acetazolamide 250 mg orally is given as a single dose 2 h prior to the scan. This is done to evaluate cerebral vascular reserve.

On the day of surgery, the patient is anesthetized in a routine fashion with midazolam, propofol, fentanyl, and rocuronium. Maintenance is with remifentanil infusion and isoflurane. Ephedrine and phenylephrine are also given during induction. After the patient is asleep, invasive monitoring including a radial artery cannulation and a triple lumen catheter are inserted. The latter is placed in the right subclavian vein.

An arterial blood gas is sent off approximately 15 min after induction. Much to everyone's surprise, the bicarbonate is 16 mEq/L with a base excess of 8.8. A repeat arterial blood gas shows the same result.

Question

What can be the cause of this severe metabolic acidosis and what will you do?

J.G. Brock-Utne, *Case Studies of Near Misses in Clinical Anesthesia*,
DOI 10.1007/978-1-4419-1179-7_76,

Solution

Acetazolamide, even in a single small dose in patients with normal kidney function, will inhibit carbonic anhydrase in the renal proximal tubule resulting in a bicarbonate diuresis and metabolic acidosis. This is often mild and self-limiting but can also be significant [1]. Often used for glaucoma and altitude sickness, the drug is also used as a single dose to evaluate cerebral vascular reserve prior to a SPECT scan [2].

In the case above [3], the acidosis was severe and prolonged. Endotracheal extubation was delayed for 48 h. There were no residual sequelae. On postoperative day 7, her bicarbonate had returned to 23 mEq/L with a base excess of 0.7.

Persistent metabolic acidosis can result in cardiovascular and CNS deficits; hence, it is critical to monitor the acid base status during the perioperative period. It is unknown why some patients have an exaggerated response to even a single dose of acetazolamide in the absence of renal pathology.

Recommendation

Remember that a single dose of acetazolamide can produce a prolonged and severe acidosis.

References

1. Heller I, Halevy J, Cohen S, Theodor E. Significant metabolic acidosis induced by acetazolamide. Arch Intern Med. 1985;145:1815–7.
2. Rim NJ, Kim HS, Shin YS, Kim SY. Which CT perfusion parameter best reflects cerebrovascular reserve? Correlation of acetazolamide-challenged CT perfusion with single-photon emission CT in Moyamoya patients. AJNR Am J Neuroradiol. 2008;29:1658–63.
3. Charles M, Kulkarni V, Brock-Utne JG. Severe metabolic acidosis during EC-IC bypass for Moyamoya, induced by acetazolamide used for a SPECT scan (a case report) (Submitted for publication 2011).

Chapter 77
Case 77: Bunionectomy Under Both General and Regional Anesthesia

A 72-year-old female (84 kg and 5 ft 8 in.), otherwise healthy, is admitted for an elective bunionectomy with osteotomy and straightening of hammertoes. The patient accepts the anesthesiologist offer of a popliteal and saphenous nerve block preoperatively for both intra- and postoperative analgesia. The block is placed under ultrasound guidance without any problems. Since the patient does not want to hear anything during the procedure, she is also given a general anesthetic with an LMA. After the surgery lasting for 2.5 h, a thick posterior plaster cast is placed. The anesthetic was uneventful and she is taken to the recovery room awake.

Thirty minutes later, she complains of severe leg pain (10/10) in the operated leg. You feel the cast and it is still warm despite the fact that it has been covered by fiberglass. The leg is lying on a pillow.

You are at a loss to understand why she should have so much pain in her leg since the block, 3.5 h ago, was perfect prior to the surgery. Fentanyl upto 150 μg over a 10-min period does not help her. Her pain is still 10/10. You decide to repeat the block. Again the block works well and the patient is now very comfortable.

Questions

Should you be pleased with your handling of this case? Is there something that you may have missed?

J.G. Brock-Utne, *Case Studies of Near Misses in Clinical Anesthesia*,
DOI 10.1007/978-1-4419-1179-7_77, © Springer Science+Business Media, LLC 2011

Solution

To your dismay, when the cast is removed on postoperative day 3, the posterior aspect of the lower leg has a nearly complete third degree burn. A skin graft is required and luckily for all concerned the patient makes a complete recovery.

When faced with such a problem in the recovery room, it is important to remember that there may be a reason for severe pain in the patient. It is prudent to call the surgeon and suggest removing and replacing the cast. If the surgeon is unwilling, you should document this fact. To repeat the regional block in these cases is not a good idea.

Clinicians should be cautious when applying a thick cast with warm dip water. A study has shown that the water to make the plaster casts should not exceed 44°C [1]. However, this will depend upon the thickness of the plaster. In a study by Halanski et al. [2], they concluded that excessive thick plaster and a dip-water temperature of >24°C should be avoided. Furthermore, the overwrapping of plaster with fiberglass should be delayed until the plaster is fully cured and cooled. Fast setting plasters have increased the risk of thermal injury [3]. Interesting prefabricated fiberglass splints appear to be safer than circumferential casts [3]. The greatest risk of thermal injury occurs when thick casts are allowed to rest on a pillow [2, 3].

Recommendation

Vigilance is always needed when evaluating a patient in the recovery room. This is especially true for a patient who has received a regional block for a surgery that necessitates a cast and now, in the recovery room, complains about large amount of pain. You must be aware of the dangers of burns associated with casts. Never repeat a regional block when you think the patient may be getting cast burn.

References

1. Read JA, Ferguson N, Ricketts DM. Plaster cast burns: the reality. Emerg Med J. 2008;25: 827–8.
2. Halanski MA, Halanski AD, Oza A, Vanderby R, Munoz A, Noonan KJ. Thermal injury with contemporary cast-application techniques and methods to circumvent morbidity. J Bone Joint Surg Am. 2007;89:2369–77.
3. Hutchinson MJ, Hutchinson MR. Factors contributing to the temperature beneath plaster of fiberglass cast material. J Orthop Surg Res. 2008;3:1–8.

Chapter 78
Case 78: Now What Would You Do?

You are a retired anesthesiologist (72" inches and 250 lb) living in Maui, Hawaii. Unfortunately, one evening, while walking on a pedestrian crossway you are hit by a bus. You roll 12 ft, sustain a concussion, a six piece comminuted humerus fracture, one fractured rib, and a 10 in. scalp laceration with lots of road burns. You are taken to the one hospital in Maui. Here, the scalp laceration is sutured. The orthopedic surgeon arrives and you inform him that you have had previous histories of difficult endotracheal intubations. He tells you not to worry as he has a very good anesthesiologist. He schedules you for a stabilization of the humerus.

Forty-eight hours later you find yourself in the operating room with the anesthesiologist. He is tall, suntanned from surfing, blond, and looks like a high school student on roller-skates. He tells you not to worry. You tell him that the last endotracheal tube (ETT), some 25 years earlier, which went through your vocal cords, was #6.0 mm. He informs you that, the only fiberoptic intubating scope in the hospital works with a #7.00 mm ETT.

You do not want a tracheostomy under local, an inhalational induction with him to "having a go," nor do you consider leaving Maui and going to Honolulu or San Francisco with a comminuted humerus fracture and a known nerve damage.

Question

Faced with this dilemma, what would you suggest should be done to access safely our anesthesiologist's airway?

J.G. Brock-Utne, *Case Studies of Near Misses in Clinical Anesthesia*,
DOI 10.1007/978-1-4419-1179-7_78, © Springer Science+Business Media, LLC 2011

Solution

This happened to a great friend of mine, Dr. Gordon Taylor, who said to the anesthesiologist: "Can we talk about the size of tube and an awake blind nasal intubation?" The young man agreed to attempt an awake blind nasal intubation with a #6.00 mm ETT. Then followed a lengthy discussion about which local anesthetic agent to be used (there is no cocaine available in Hawaii) and which vasoconstrictor agent. The conversation ended with Gordon saying "Maybe we could do it together?" The young man reluctantly agreed. The fibreoptic scope with the #7.00 mm ETT was to be held in reserve. Through the IV the young man gave Gordon glycopyrrolate 0.2 mg and meperidine 50 mg. Lidocaine 5% ointment was used to grease the right nostril. With an atomizer, lidocaine and afrin (oxymetazoline hydrochloride 0.05%) were administrated to the posterior pharynx and cords. Gordon tells the rest of the story like this: "As the young man advanced the ETT through my right nostril, I slowed him down a bit and asked to advance the ETT myself. I felt the tip of the ETT on the cords and gave it a little push. The last thing I remember was a female voice whispering: 'He intubated himself'."

Gordon obviously survived to tell the story, and hopes for a 90% recovery of his neural injury 18 months after the accident.

Awake blind nasal intubations are rarely being taught today. In Gordon's time as a resident in 1960 at the Westminster hospital in London, England it was a very popular. The prevailing intubation technique for dental surgery was blind nasal intubation. To make the intubation easier with large tidal volumes carbon dioxide gas was added to the anesthesia mixture. The CO_2 had its own rotatometer placed beside the oxygen and nitrous oxide. On the back of the machine there was CO_2 cylinder.

The author, JGBU, recalls that in South Africa we did not have CO_2 gas available. To get a similar effect as CO_2, ether was used after the patient was asleep with halothane. Ether made the respiration slow and with a large tidal volume. We also had a little whistle that we attached to the proximal end of the ETT. In this way everyone in the room could hear that the patient was intubated safely. It was also very interesting to note how quiet the operating room became prior to the successful ETT placement.

It is our opinion (Gordon and I) that it is a pity that for various reasons, the next generation of anesthesiologist are not taught or encouraged the use of awake blind nasal intubation.

Recommendation

Difficult endotracheal intubation remains a classic challenge for any anesthesia provider. To keep the patient breathing while getting control of the airway is by far the safest thing to do. This is especially true when you, as the patient, are aware of all the problems associated with a difficult intubation. Dr. Gordon Taylor is an example.

Chapter 79
Case 79: A Strange Case

A 45-year-old female (70 kg and 5 ft 11 in.) is admitted as an outpatient for laparoscopy for endometriosis under general anesthesia. You see her in the preoperative area with her husband. She tells you she has not had any previous operations and is very healthy. She denies any allergies. Reading the outpatient note, you see that she has had a chin implant. When you ask her again she says that is a mistake.

You place an IV and sedate her with midazolam IV and take her back to the operating room. Here you place routine noninvasive monitors. The case is scheduled for 3 h. You induce a routine general anesthetic with propofol, fentanyl, and rocuronium. Maintenance is with nitrous oxide in 30% oxygen and sevoflurane and morphine. After 30 min the surgeon says he is finished. To judge her neuromuscular blocking status, you place two electrodes on the side of her forehead, above and below the angle of the eye. Train of four, double-burst and titanic stimulation patterns are tried at maximum current output but no visible evoked contractions are seen in the orbicularis oculi. You try the nerve stimulator on your ulnar nerve at the wrist and discover that it works very well, even at very low current output.

Questions

What will you do? Wait for the rocuronium to wear off, look for other causes of prolonged block, or give reversal?

J.G. Brock-Utne, *Case Studies of Near Misses in Clinical Anesthesia*,
DOI 10.1007/978-1-4419-1179-7_79, © Springer Science+Business Media, LLC 2011

Solution

You certainly do not want to give reversal in a patient who is potentially fully paralyzed. Neostigmine will potentially accentuate the neuromuscular block.

You place the electrodes over the patient's ulnar nerve at the wrist. A train-of-four stimulus provokes four forceful and fade-free muscle contractions. The patient enjoys an uncomplicated emergence from anesthesia [1]. Later she admits (without her husband present) to have had Botox injections to have her face and chin implant.

We also had a case where we were unaware that the patient, a TV announcer, had a chin implant making the endotracheal intubation a nightmare [2]. All went well though.

Recommendation

In patients who may have had plastic surgery with Botox injection, use the ulnar nerve when possible to monitor neuromuscular function.

References

1. Ward SJ, Harrop-Griffiths W. Botox injections and monitoring neuromuscular blockade. Anaesthesia. 2006;61:714–26.
2. Brock-Utne JG, Brodsky JB, Haddow GR, Azar DR, Kaye B. Difficult laryngoscopy masked by previous cosmetic surgery. Plast Reconstr Surg. 1991;87:1143–4.

Chapter 80
Case 80: A Chronic Pain Patient

Today you are scheduled to anesthetize a 29-year-old female (5 ft 8 in. and 70 kg) for reimplantation of ureters into the bladder. She has had multiple urological surgeries after a failed one 5 years ago. She is a chronic pain patient on the usual medication including fentanyl patch. You see her for the first time in the preoperative area. Her heart rate is 86 bpm, BP 145/85, and respiratory rate 30. She complains about severe abdominal pain (10/10). Her mum and dad, who are at the bedside, inform you that this is her usual pain level, only today it seems worse. The patient agrees but tells you that she has not taken any of her usual pain medication this morning except for the fentanyl patch. She has been fasting since midnight. The patient requests IV pain medication before you take her back to the operating room.

Question

Is there anything else you would like to do before you give her sedation and/or analgesia?

J.G. Brock-Utne, *Case Studies of Near Misses in Clinical Anesthesia*,
DOI 10.1007/978-1-4419-1179-7_80, © Springer Science+Business Media, LLC 2011

Solution

Examine the patient and also her abdomen. This case happened to us. In this case we diagnosed an acute abdomen caused by the combination of fecal impaction and bowel prep. We canceled the case and the surgeon was thankful. The fecal impaction was treated and the surgery undertaken at a later date.

We must consider ourselves lucky. It would have been very easy to give the patient sedation and analgesia without examining the patient's abdomen. Then with the patient more comfortable, take her to operating room and anesthetize her.

Always remember to examine your patient. It is a sad fact that, it would seem that in the modern medical profession, physical exam is often not used or encouraged [1].

Recommendation

Always examine your patient. You will be thankful you did.

Reference

1. Jauhar S. The demise of the physical exam. N Engl J Med. 2006;354:548–51.

Index

J.G. Brock-Utne, *Case Studies of Near Misses in Clinical Anesthesia*,
DOI 10.1007/978-1-4419-1179-7, © Springer Science+Business Media, LLC 2011

K

L

M

N

O